HISTOLOGICAL TYPING OF
UPPER RESPIRATORY TRACT TUMOURS

HISTOLOGICAL TYPING OF UPPER RESPIRATORY TRACT TUMOURS

K. SHANMUGARATNAM

*Head, WHO International Reference Centre for the Histological Classification
of Upper Respiratory Tract Tumours, Department of Pathology, University of Singapore*

in collaboration with

L. H. SOBIN

*Pathologist,
World Health Organization,
Geneva, Switzerland*

·and pathologists in 10 countries

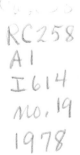

WORLD HEALTH ORGANIZATION

GENEVA

1978

LIST OF PARTICIPANTS

WHO International Reference Centre for the Histological Classification of Upper Respiratory Tract Tumours,[1] Department of Pathology, University of Singapore

Head of Centre

Dr K. SHANMUGARATNAM

Participants

Dr W. C. BAUER, Division of Surgical Pathology, Barnes Hospital, St Louis, MO, USA

Dr S. C. BESUSCHIO, Academia Nacional de Medicina de Buenos Aires, Buenos Aires, Argentina

Dr M. CAMMOUN, Institute Salah Azaiz, Tunis, Tunisia

Dr. I. FRIEDMANN, Northwick Park Hospital, Harrow, Middlesex, England

Dr. V. HYAMS, Armed Forces Institute of Pathology, Washington, DC, USA

Dr O. KLEINSASSER, University Ear, Nose and Throat Clinic, Marburg-Lahn, Federal Republic of Germany

Dr N. I. KOLYCHEVA, Oncological and Radiological Research Institute, Alma Ata, Kazakhstan, USSR

Dr. L. H. SOBIN, Cancer, World Health Organization, Geneva, Switzerland

Reviewers

Dr N. F. C. GOWING, Department of Pathology, Royal Marsden Hospital, London, England

Dr C. MICHEAU, Institut Gustave-Roussy, Villejuif, France

Dr M. DAOIZ MENDOZA, Department of Pathology, Faculty of Medicine, Montevideo, Uruguay

Dr G. MOBERGER, Department of Pathology, Radiumhemmet, Stockholm, Sweden

Dr R. RAICHEV, Department of Pathology, Oncological Research Institute, Sofia, Bulgaria

---

[1] Following a decision taken by the World Health Organization in 1974 in the interest of uniformity, all WHO-designated centres have been renamed WHO Collaborating Centres; thus the above centre is now known as the WHO Collaborating Centre for the Histological Classification of Upper Respiratory Tract Tumours.

The photomicrographs reproduced in this volume were taken by Mr Tan Tee Chok, Department of Pathology, University of Singapore.

CONTENTS

Colour photomicrographs

GENERAL PREFACE TO THE SERIES

Among the prerequisites for comparative studies of cancer are international agreement on histological criteria for the classification of cancer types and a standardized nomenclature. At present, pathologists use different terms for the same pathological entity, and furthermore the same term is sometimes applied to lesions of different types. An internationally agreed classification of tumours, acceptable alike to physicians, surgeons, radiologists, pathologists and statisticians, would enable cancer workers in all parts of the world to compare their findings and would facilitate collaboration among them.

In a report published in 1952,[1] a subcommittee of the WHO Expert Committee on Health Statistics discussed the general principles that should govern the statistical classification of tumours and agreed that, to ensure the necessary flexibility and ease in coding, three separate classifications were needed according to (1) anatomical site, (2) histological type, and (3) degree of malignancy. A classification according to anatomical site is available in the International Classification of Diseases.[2]

The question of establishing a universally accepted classification by histological type has received much attention during the last 20 years and a particularly valuable Atlas of Tumor Pathology—*already numbering more than 40 volumes—is being published in the USA by the Armed Forces Institute of Pathology under the auspices of the National Research Council. An* Illustrated Tumour Nomenclature *in English, French, German, Latin, Russian and Spanish has also been published by the International Union Against Cancer (UICC).*

In 1956 the WHO Executive Board passed a resolution[3] requesting the Director-General to explore the possibility that WHO might organize centres in various parts of the world and arrange for the collection of human tissues and their histological classification. The main purpose of such centres would be to develop histological definitions of cancer types and to facilitate the wide adoption of a uniform nomenclature. This resolution was endorsed by the Tenth World Health Assembly in May 1957[4] and the following month a Study Group on Histological Classification of Cancer Types met in Oslo to

---

[1] *Wld Hlth Org. techn. Rep. Ser.*, 1952, No. 53, p. 45.

[2] World Health Organization (1967) *Manual of the International Statistical Classification of Diseases, Injuries, and Causes of Death*, 1965 revision, Geneva.

[3] *Off. Rec. Wld Hlth Org.*, 1956, **68**, 14 (Resolution EB17.R.40).

[4] *Off. Rec. Wld Hlth Org.*, 1957, **79**, 467 (Resolution WHA10.18).

advise WHO on its implementation. The Group recommended criteria for selecting tumour sites for study and suggested a procedure for the drafting of histological classifications and testing their validity. Briefly, the procedure is as follows:

For each tumour site, a tentative histopathological typing and classification is drawn up by a group of experts, consisting of up to ten pathologists working in the field in question. An international reference centre and a number of collaborating laboratories are then designated by WHO to evaluate the proposed classification. These laboratories exchange histological preparations, accompanied by clinical information. The histological typing is then made in accordance with the proposed classification. Subsequently, one or more technical meetings are called by WHO to facilitate an exchange of opinions and the classification is amended to take account of criticisms.

In addition to preparing the publication and the photomicrographs for it, the reference centre produces up to 100 sets of microscope slides showing the major histological types for distribution to national societies of pathology.

Since 1958, WHO has established 23 centres covering tumours of the lung; breast; soft tissues; oropharynx; bone; ovaries; salivary glands; thyroid; skin; male urogenital tract; jaws; female genital tract; stomach and oesophagus; intestines; central nervous system; liver, biliary tract and pancreas; upper respiratory tract; eye; and endocrine glands; as well as oral precancerous conditions; the leukaemias and lymphomas; comparative oncology; and exfoliative cytology. This work has involved more than 300 pathologists from over 50 countries. A number of these centres have completed their work, and most of their classifications have already been published (see page 6).

The World Health Organization is indebted to the many pathologists who have participated and are participating in this large undertaking. The pioneer work of many other international and national organizations in the field of histological classification of tumours has greatly facilitated the task undertaken by WHO. Particular gratitude is expressed to the National Cancer Institute, USA, which, through the National Research Council and the USA National Committee for the International Council of Societies of Pathology, is providing financial support to accelerate this work. Finally, WHO wishes to record its appreciation of the valuable help it has received from the International Council of Societies of Pathology (ICSP) in proposing participants and in undertaking to distribute copies of the classifications, with corresponding sets of microscope slides, to national societies of pathology all over the world.

PREFACE TO HISTOLOGICAL TYPING
OF UPPER RESPIRATORY TRACT TUMOURS

The WHO International Reference Centre for the Histological Classification of Upper Respiratory Tract Tumours was established in 1972 at the Department of Pathology, University of Singapore.

The Centre distributed histological sections from selected cases to the participants, a list of which will be found on page 5, for typing according to a tentative classification drawn up at a WHO consultation in 1972. In all, 320 cases were thus studied and were reviewed at meetings in 1974 and 1975 attended by the participants. The classification, its definitions, and its nomenclature were amended at these meetings in the light of this study. The classification and selected cases were reviewed by a second group of pathologists designated by WHO (see page 5). At the meeting in 1975 the present classification was adopted.

It will, of course, be appreciated that the classification reflects the present state of knowledge, and modifications are almost certain to be needed as experience accumulates. Although the present classification has been adopted by the members of the group, it necessarily represents a view from which some pathologists may wish to dissent. It is nevertheless hoped that, in the interests of international cooperation, all pathologists will try to use the classification as put forward. Criticisms and suggestions for its improvement will be welcomed. These should be sent to the World Health Organization, Geneva, Switzerland.

The publications in the series International Histological Classification of Tumours *are not intended to serve as textbooks but rather to promote the adoption of a uniform terminology and categorization of tumours that will facilitate and improve communication among cancer workers. For this reason the literature references have intentionally been kept to a minimum, and readers are referred to standard works on the subject for extensive bibliographies.*

INTRODUCTION

This volume deals with tumours arising from the following sites:

the nasal cavity and paranasal sinuses;

the nasopharynx;

the larynx, hypopharynx, and trachea;

the external ear; and

the middle and inner ear.

Most of these sites are relatively inaccessible, and biopsy materials are often obtained by forceps removal or curettage. The tissue samples received by the pathologist are often small and may not be fully representative of the lesion. Furthermore, the method of obtaining specimens may cause artefactual traumatic distortion of the tissues. The histological appearances may also be complicated by ulceration and secondary inflammatory reaction. It is therefore important to make allowance for these changes when examining biopsy specimens from these sites.

The classification

This classification is based primarily on the histological characteristics of the tumours and is therefore concerned with morphologically identifiable cell types and histological patterns as seen with conventional light microscopy. Although many of the histological terms and definitions used may have histogenetic implications, this classification is not based on histogenesis.

The tumour types listed in this classification are those that occur either specifically or commonly in the sites comprising the upper respiratory tract and ear. The classification of tumours arising from each of these sites is given separately. However, as the same tumour type may occur in more than one anatomical site, the definitions and illustrations have been grouped together.

The upper respiratory tract comprises a wide variety of epithelial, glandular, lymphoid, connective tissue, and bony elements. It is not surprising, therefore, that the tumours occurring in this area include several types that have been defined and illustrated in previous volumes in this series. These will be described in summary form.

Terminology

The term " tumour " is used synonymously with neoplasm. The phrase " tumour-like " is applied to lesions which clinically or morphologically resemble neoplasms but do not behave biologically in a neoplastic manner. They are included in this classification because they are often confused with tumours and because of the ill-defined borderline between some neoplasms and certain non-neoplastic lesions. Time-honoured terms have generally been retained. Synonyms are included only if they have been widely used or if they are considered to be helpful in the understanding of the lesions. In such cases, the preferred terms are given first, followed by the synonyms within brackets.

Grading of tumours

Qualifying phrases are widely used to indicate the degree of differentiation of certain types of tumours. Although this aspect has been considered of prognostic value in certain cases, it may be of doubtful value in others. The grading of certain types of malignant tumours by the use of modifying phrases to indicate the degree of differentiation is widely practised. This deserves continuing investigation in relation to all types. It is recommended that the following categories be used, particularly when dealing with carcinomas:

Well differentiated—a carcinoma with histological and cellular features that closely resemble normal epithelium of similar type.

Moderately differentiated—a carcinoma with histological features intermediate between well differentiated and poorly differentiated.

Poorly differentiated—a carcinoma with histological and cellular features which only barely resemble normal epithelium of similar type.

Carcinomas may contain areas with different degrees of differentiation. It has been postulated that the biological behaviour of a tumour is a reflection of its most poorly differentiated components, and such tumours should be graded on this basis. Tumour biopsies from the growing edges of the tumour or from portions directly adjacent to ulcerative or inflammatory processes are not suitable for purposes of grading.

It must be emphasized that factors other than histological grade influence the behaviour of tumours and prognosis. Special consideration should be given to the stage or extent of tumour at the time of diagnosis, the patterns of growth and spread of the tumour, and the immunological responses of the patient. The accessibility of the tumour and involvement of cranial bones are particularly important in tumours of the upper respiratory tract. Interference with respiration, secondary infection, and pulmonary involvement are also important considerations.

HISTOLOGICAL CLASSIFICATION OF TUMOURS OF THE NASAL CAVITY AND PARANASAL SINUSES (EXCLUDING NASAL VESTIBULE)

I. EPITHELIAL TUMOURS

A. BENIGN

1. Squamous cell papilloma (1) *

2. " Transitional " papilloma [cylindric cell papilloma, respiratory epithelial papilloma] (3)

   (a) inverted

   (b) exophytic

3. Adenoma (4)

4. Oxyphilic adenoma [oncocytoma] (5)

5. Pleomorphic adenoma [mixed tumour] (6)

B. MALIGNANT

1. Squamous cell carcinoma (9)

2. Verrucous (squamous) carcinoma (10)

3. Spindle cell (squamous) carcinoma (11)

4. " Transitional " carcinoma [cylindric cell carcinoma, nonkeratinizing carcinoma, respiratory epithelial carcinoma] (12)

5. Adenocarcinoma (16)

6. Mucinous adenocarcinoma (17)

7. Adenoid cystic carcinoma (18)

---

* The numbers in parentheses refer to paragraphs in the definitions and explanatory notes.

8. Mucoepidermoid carcinoma (19)

9. Others (21)

10. Undifferentiated carcinoma (22)

II. SOFT TISSUE TUMOURS (23)

A. BENIGN

1. Haemangioma (26)

2. Haemangiopericytoma (27)

3. Neurofibroma (31)

4. Neurilemmoma [schwannoma] (32)

5. Myxoma (33)

6. Fibroxanthoma [fibrous histiocytoma] (34)

7. Others

B. MALIGNANT

1. Malignant haemangiopericytoma (27)

2. Fibrosarcoma (36)

3. Rhabdomyosarcoma (37)

4. Neurogenic sarcoma [neurofibrosarcoma and malignant schwannoma] (40)

5. Malignant fibroxanthoma [malignant fibrous histiocytoma] (41)

6. Others

III. TUMOURS OF BONE AND CARTILAGE (42)

A. BENIGN

1. Chondroma (43)

2. Osteoma (44)

3. Ossifying fibroma (45)

4. Others

B. MALIGNANT

    1. Chondrosarcoma (46)

    2. Osteosarcoma (47)

    3. Others

IV. TUMOURS OF LYMPHOID AND HAEMATOPOIETIC TISSUES

    1. Malignant lymphomas (48)

        (*a*) Lymphosarcoma

        (*b*) Burkitt's tumour

        (*c*) Reticulosarcoma

        (*d*) Plasmacytoma (49)

        (*e*) Hodgkin's disease

V. MISCELLANEOUS TUMOURS

A. BENIGN

    1. Teratoma (50)

    2. Meningioma (52)

    3. Odontogenic tumours (53)

    4. Melanotic neuroectodermal tumour [melanotic progonoma] (54)

    5. Others

B. MALIGNANT

    1. Malignant melanoma (55)

    2. Olfactory neurogenic [esthesioneurogenic] tumours (56)

    3. Others

VI. SECONDARY TUMOURS

VII. UNCLASSIFIED TUMOURS

VIII. TUMOUR-LIKE LESIONS

1. Pseudoepitheliomatous hyperplasia (59)

2. Oncocytic metaplasia and hyperplasia (65)

3. Cysts (66)

4. Mucocele (67)

5. Angiogranuloma [" haemangioma " of granulation tissue type, granuloma pyogenicum] (68)

6. Nasal polyp (70)

7. Fibromatosis (74)

8. Fibrous dysplasia (75)

9. Giant cell " reparative " granuloma (76)

10. Infective granulomas (78)

11. Cholesterol granuloma (79)

12. Lethal midline granuloma [Stewart's granuloma, " malignant " granuloma] (82)

13. Wegener's granulomatosis (83)

14. Nasal glial heterotopia [nasal " glioma "] (85)

15. Meningocele/meningo-encephalocele (86)

HISTOLOGICAL CLASSIFICATION OF TUMOURS OF THE NASOPHARYNX

I. EPITHELIAL TUMOURS

A. BENIGN

1. Squamous cell papilloma (1)

2. Oxyphilic adenoma [oncocytoma] (5)

3. Pleomorphic adenoma [mixed tumour] (6)

4. Others

B. MALIGNANT

1. Nasopharyngeal carcinoma (13)

   (*a*) Squamous cell carcinoma [keratinizing squamous cell carcinoma]

   (*b*) Non-keratinizing carcinoma

   (*c*) Undifferentiated carcinoma [undifferentiated carcinoma of nasopharyngeal type]

2. Adenocarcinoma (16)

3. Adenoid cystic carcinoma (18)

4. Others

II. SOFT TISSUE TUMOURS

A. BENIGN

1. Juvenile angiofibroma (25)

2. Neurofibroma (31)

    3. Neurilemmoma [schwannoma] (32)

    4. Paraganglioma [chemodectoma] (35)

    5. Others

B. MALIGNANT

    1. Fibrosarcoma (36)

    2. Rhabdomyosarcoma (37)

    3. Neurogenic sarcoma [neurofibrosarcoma, malignant schwannoma] (40)

    4. Others

III. TUMOURS OF BONE AND CARTILAGE (42)

IV. TUMOURS OF LYMPHOID AND HAEMATOPOIETIC TISSUES

    1. Malignant lymphomas (48)
        (*a*) Lymphosarcoma
        (*b*) Burkitt's tumour
        (*c*) Reticulosarcoma
        (*d*) Plasmacytoma (49)
        (*e*) Hodgkin's disease

V. MISCELLANEOUS TUMOURS

A. BENIGN

    1. Teratoma (50)
        (*a*) solid
        (*b*) cystic [dermoid cyst]

    2. Pituitary adenoma (51)

    3. Meningioma (52)

    4. Others

B. MALIGNANT

    1. Malignant melanoma (55)

    2. Chordoma (57)

    3. Craniopharyngioma (58)

    4. Others

VI. SECONDARY TUMOURS

VII. UNCLASSIFIED TUMOURS

VIII. TUMOUR-LIKE LESIONS

1. Pseudoepitheliomatous hyperplasia (59)

2. Oncocytic metaplasia and hyperplasia (65)

3. Cysts (66)

4. Angiogranuloma [" haemangioma " of granulation tissue type, granuloma pyogenicum] (68)

5. Fibromatosis (74)

6. Amyloid deposits (77)

7. Infective granulomas (78)

8. Benign lymphoid hyperplasia [" adenoids "] (81)

9. Lethal midline granuloma [Stewart's granuloma, " malignant " granuloma] (82)

10. Wegener's granulomatosis (83)

HISTOLOGICAL CLASSIFICATION OF TUMOURS OF THE LARYNX, HYPOPHARYNX, AND TRACHEA

I. EPITHELIAL TUMOURS

A. BENIGN

    1. Squamous cell papilloma/papillomatosis (2)

    2. Oxyphilic adenoma [oncocytoma] (5)

    3. Others

B. MALIGNANT

    1. Carcinoma in situ [intraepithelial carcinoma] (8)

    2. Squamous cell carcinoma (9)

    3. Verrucous (squamous) carcinoma (10)

    4. Spindle cell (squamous) carcinoma (11)

    5. Adenocarcinoma (16)

    6. Adenoid cystic carcinoma (18)

    7. Carcinoid tumour (20)

    8. Others

    9. Undifferentiated carcinoma (22)

II. SOFT TISSUE TUMOURS (23)

A. BENIGN

    1. Lipoma (24)

    2. Haemangioma (26)

    3. Leiomyoma (28)

4. Rhabdomyoma (29)

5. Granular cell tumour (30)

6. Neurofibroma (31)

7. Neurilemmoma [schwannoma] (32)

8. Paraganglioma [chemodectoma] (35)

9. Others

B. MALIGNANT

1. Fibrosarcoma (36)

2. Rhabdomyosarcoma (37)

3. Angiosarcoma (38)

4. Kaposi's sarcoma (39)

5. Others

III. TUMOURS OF BONE AND CARTILAGE (42)

A. BENIGN

1. Chondroma (43)

2. Others

B. MALIGNANT

1. Chondrosarcoma (46)

2. Others

IV. TUMOURS OF LYMPHOID AND HAEMATOPOIETIC TISSUES

V. MISCELLANEOUS TUMOURS

VI. SECONDARY TUMOURS

VII. UNCLASSIFIED TUMOURS

VIII. TUMOUR-LIKE LESIONS

1. Pseudoepitheliomatous hyperplasia (59)

2. Epithelial abnormalities (62)
   (*a*) Keratosis/hyperplasia [keratosis without atypia] (63)
   (*b*) Dysplasia [keratosis with atypia] (64)

3. Oncocytic metaplasia and hyperplasia (65)

4. Cysts (66)

5. Intubation granuloma/" contact " ulcer (69)

6. Vocal cord polyps (71)
   (*a*) fibrous
   (*b*) vascular
   (*c*) hyalinized
   (*d*) myxoid

7. Amyloid deposits (77)

8. Infective granulomas (78)

9. Plasma cell granuloma (80)

10. Lethal midline granuloma [Stewart's granuloma, " malignant " granuloma] (82)

11. Wegener's granulomatosis (83)

12. Tracheopathia osteochondroplastica (87)

HISTOLOGICAL CLASSIFICATION OF TUMOURS OF THE EXTERNAL EAR (PINNA AND EXTERNAL AUDITORY MEATUS)

I. EPITHELIAL TUMOURS

A. BENIGN

    1. Squamous cell papilloma (1)

    2. Ceruminous adenoma (15)

    3. Others

B. MALIGNANT

    1. Squamous cell carcinoma (9)

    2. Basal cell carcinoma (14)

    3. Ceruminous adenocarcinoma (15)

    4. Adenoid cystic carcinoma (18)

    5. Others

II. SOFT TISSUE TUMOURS

A. BENIGN

    1. Haemangioma (26)

    2. Neurofibroma (31)

    3. Neurilemmoma [schwannoma] (32)

    4. Others

B. MALIGNANT

    1. Fibrosarcoma (36)

2. Rhabdomyosarcoma (37)

3. Others

III. TUMOURS OF BONE AND CARTILAGE (42)

A. BENIGN

1. Chondroma (43)

2. Osteoma (44)

3. Others

B. MALIGNANT

1. Chondrosarcoma (46)

2. Osteosarcoma (47)

3. Others

IV. MISCELLANEOUS TUMOURS

V. SECONDARY TUMOURS

VI. UNCLASSIFIED TUMOURS

VII. TUMOUR-LIKE LESIONS

1. Keratosis obturans (60)

2. Otic [aural] polyp (72)

3. Keloid (73)

4. Chondrodermatitis nodularis chronica helicis (88)

HISTOLOGICAL CLASSIFICATION OF TUMOURS OF THE MIDDLE AND INNER EAR

I. EPITHELIAL TUMOURS

A. BENIGN

    1. Adenoma (4)

    2. Others

B. MALIGNANT

    1. Squamous cell carcinoma (9)

    2. Others

II. SOFT TISSUE TUMOURS (23)

A. BENIGN

    1. Neurofibroma (31)

    2. Neurilemmoma [schwannoma] (32)

    3. Paraganglioma [glomus jugulare tumour, chemodectoma] (35)

    4. Others

B. MALIGNANT

    1. Malignant paraganglioma [malignant glomus jugulare tumour, malignant chemodectoma] (35)

    2. Rhabdomyosarcoma (37)

    3. Neurogenic sarcoma (40)

    4. Others

III. TUMOURS OF BONE AND CARTILAGE (42)

A. BENIGN

    1. Osteoma (44)

    2. Others

B. MALIGNANT

    1. Chondrosarcoma (46)

    2. Osteosarcoma (47)

    3. Others

IV. MISCELLANEOUS TUMOURS

A. BENIGN

    1. Meningioma (50)

    2. Others

B. MALIGNANT

V. SECONDARY TUMOURS

VI. UNCLASSIFIED TUMOURS

VII. TUMOUR-LIKE LESIONS

    1. Epidermoid " cholesteatoma " (61)

    2. Otic [aural] polyp (72)

    3. Fibrous dysplasia (75)

    4. Cholesterol granuloma (79)

    5. Histiocytosis X (84)

    6. Tympanosclerosis (89)

DEFINITIONS AND EXPLANATORY NOTES

EPITHELIAL TUMOURS

1. *Squamous cell papilloma* (Fig. 1): A benign epithelial neoplasm formed of stratified squamous epithelium.

These tumours are usually exophytic. They consist of a thickened layer of well-differentiated stratified squamous epithelium covering arborescent stalks of vascular connective tissue. Intercellular bridges and/or varying degrees of keratinization are present. In the upper respiratory tract this neoplasm may occur not only in areas normally lined by stratified squamous epithelium but also in areas normally lined by ciliated columnar epithelium.

2. *Squamous cell papilloma/papillomatosis of the larynx* (Fig. 2): A benign epithelial neoplasm formed of stratified squamous epithelium.

Two main forms of squamous cell papilloma are recognized clinically in the larynx—a *juvenile* type that is usually multiple (papillomatosis) and an *adult* type that is usually single. These types are histologically indistinguishable. The papillomas show branching fibrovascular stalks covered by a thickened layer of well-differentiated stratified squamous epithelium that is often parakeratotic on its surface. Mitoses may be present. Focal keratosis is common; mucous and ciliated cells are occasionally present.

Laryngeal papillomas seldom become malignant. Juvenile papillomas often undergo spontaneous involution. Malignant change may develop in irradiated juvenile papillomas. The presence of epithelial dysplasia in adult papillomas or in squamous cell papillomatosis should be regarded with a suspicion of malignancy; however, only a small number of non-irradiated adult papillomas become malignant.

A rare form of squamous cell papillomatosis occurs in which there is progressive involvement of the upper and lower respiratory tract including the lung.

3. " *Transitional* " *papilloma* [cylindric cell papilloma, respiratory epithelial papilloma] (Fig. 3–8): A benign epithelial tumour of nasal respiratory epithelium. Areas of well-differentiated columnar, even ciliated, epithelium may be present, as may varying gradations of squamous differentiation.

These tumours are generally polypoid. They may be further classified into *inverted* papillomas, in which the epithelial elements exhibit invaginations into the stroma, and *exophytic* papillomas, which exhibit a fungiform or papillary structure. In general, inverted papillomas arise from the lateral walls of the nasal cavity and exophytic papillomas from the surfaces of the nasal septum. The majority of papillomas are unilateral and have a tendency to recur.

Transitional papillomas are usually of the *inverted* type. These tumours are commonly found in the nasal cavity and in the paranasal sinuses and are rare in other parts of the upper respiratory tract. The infolding of the mucosa in the inverted papilloma may give a superficial impression, in section, of an invasive epithelial growth in which cell masses with central degeneration appear to lie deep to the surface of the tumour. The basement membrane, however, is intact and continuous with that of the remainder of the surface epithelium. There may be transition from cylindrical to squamous cell type. The nuclei in the basal layer may show some irregularity with hyperchromatism but the cellular arrangement is generally regular and there is no gross disturbance of polarity. Although these tumours do not arise from transitional epithelium, the widely used term " transitional " papilloma has been retained.

Also included in this category are papillary tumours lined by pseudostratified respiratory epithelium containing mucus-filled microcysts. They are typically exophytic and have been referred to as *columnar cell papillomas*.

4. *Adenoma* (Fig. 9–10): A benign epithelial tumour forming glandular structures.

Adenomas of the nasal cavity and paranasal sinuses may assume compact, tubular, papillary, and/or cystic forms. This category includes monomorphic adenomas of the salivary type.

5. *Oxyphilic adenoma* [oncocytoma] (Fig. 11): A benign tumour of adenomatous morphology composed of large cuboidal or columnar cells characterized by distinctive granular eosinophilic cytoplasm.

The characteristic tumour cells may be arranged in compact sheets or cords, or in tubular or papillary structures. A bilayered appearance may be present. In the larynx the lesion may assume a cystic form. The distinction between an oxyphilic neoplasm and oncocytic metaplasia is often difficult (see para. 65).

6. *Pleomorphic adenoma* [mixed tumour] (Fig. 12): A circumscribed tumour characterized microscopically by its pleomorphic or " mixed " appearance with clearly recognizable epithelial tissue intermingled with tissue of mucoid, myxoid, or chondroid appearance. The epithelial components may take the form of ducts, sheets of myoepithelial cells, or squamous structures.

7. *Adenoma of the middle ear* (Fig. 13): An epithelial tumour of apparently benign behaviour occurring in the middle ear and histologically revealing an adenomatous morphology with occasional areas of uniform sheet-like cells.

It has been suggested that this tumour may originate from middle ear mucosa. The neoplasm has an adenomatous, occasionally papillary, pattern. Large sheet-like areas of tumour cells may be present but in every case an adenomatous element can be found. Pleomorphism may be present but mitotic activity is absent. Mucin production may be demonstrated.

8. *Carcinoma in situ* [intraepithelial carcinoma] (Fig. 14–15). A lesion in which the entire thickness of the epithelium shows malignant cytological features, with loss of polarity or loss of normal stratification but without evidence of stromal invasion.

9. *Squamous cell carcinoma* (Fig. 16–17): A malignant epithelial tumour with evidence of squamous differentiation.

Squamous cell carcinomas of the upper respiratory tract exhibit the same range of histological appearances as those arising in other sites. The presence of intercellular bridges and keratinization are obvious in well-differentiated neoplasms. These features are barely evident in the poorly differentiated carcinomas.

10. *Verrucous (squamous) carcinoma* (Fig. 18–19): A warty variant of squamous cell carcinoma, characterized by a pronounced overgrowth of well-differentiated keratinizing epithelium thrown up into regular vertical folds.

Vertical sections of the neoplasm show epithelial spires capped by a thick parakeratotic or keratotic layer. Bulbous acanthotic folds push into the submucosal tissues, in which there is a heavy inflammatory reaction. Mitoses are rare and the usual cytological appearance of the epithelial cells is quite bland. These benign cellular features and the orderly maturation sequence belie the local destructive nature of the tumour. However, it should be recognized that small focal areas of cellular atypia may be found as a minor component of a large lesion.

The tumour is slow-growing and often involves an extensive area. It tends to invade local structures but lacks the ability to metastasize. Biopsy material from superficial areas may not show the characteristic histological features. The verrucous carcinoma is distinguished from well-differentiated squamous cell carcinoma by its minimal atypia, its growth pattern, and the absence of metastases.

11. *Spindle cell (squamous) carcinoma* (Fig. 20–22): A variant of squamous cell carcinoma with a biphasic appearance due to the presence of a component that is identifiable as a squamous cell carcinoma and a spindle cell component derived from it.

The spindle cell component has a sarcoma-like growth pattern. It often exhibits marked cellular pleomorphism and abnormal mitoses. It is frequently admixed with nonneoplastic connective tissue elements. The component that is obviously squamous may be quite inconspicuous. Areas of transition of the squamous cell carcinoma into the spindle cell component are demonstrable and provide evidence that the tumour is a variant of squamous cell carcinoma. The tumour, when present in the larynx and hypopharynx, is generally polypoid and ulcerated. Tumours in the nasopharynx, nasal cavity, and paranasal sinuses are usually fungating. Spindle cell carcinoma has been referred to as *pleomorphic carcinoma* and *pseudosarcoma*.

12. *" Transitional" carcinoma* [cylindric cell carcinoma, non-keratinizing carcinoma, respiratory epithelial carcinoma] (Fig. 23–24): A malignant tumour composed of cells of respiratory epithelial type.

In many areas the tumour is intraepithelial with an intact basement membrane. In the invasive areas, the tumour cells may form ribbon-like bands. The overall growth pattern is typically one of *en bloc* invasion with a " pushing border ". Foci of squamous metaplasia may occur. Although these tumours do not arise from transitional epithelium, the widely used term " transitional " carcinoma has been retained.

13. *Nasopharyngeal carcinoma* (Fig. 25–34): A malignant tumour of the epithelium lining the surface and crypts of the nasopharynx.

On the basis of electron microscopic findings, all types of nasopharyngeal carcinoma may be regarded as variants of squamous cell carcinoma. These tumours may be classified into the following groups according to their predominant pattern on light microscopy.

(*a*) *Squamous cell carcinoma* [keratinizing squamous cell carcinoma] (Fig. 25–26). A nasopharyngeal carcinoma showing definite evidence of squamous differentiation with the presence of intercellular bridges and/or keratinization over most of its extent. It may be graded as well, moderately, or poorly differentiated (see p. 14).

(*b*) *Nonkeratinizing carcinoma* (Fig. 27–29). A nasopharyngeal carcinoma showing evidence of differentiation with a maturation sequence that results in cells in which squamous differentiation is not evident on light microscopy. The tumour cells have fairly well defined cell margins and show an arrangement that is stratified or pavemented and not syncytial. A plexiform pattern is common. Some tumours may exhibit a clear cell structure due to the presence of cytoplasmic glycogen. There is no evidence of mucin production or of glandular differentiation.

(*c*) *Undifferentiated carcinoma* [undifferentiated carcinoma of nasopharyngeal type] (Fig. 30–34). The tumour cells have oval or round vesicular nuclei and prominent nucleoli. The cell margins are indistinct and the tumour exhibits a syncytial rather than pavemented appearance. Spindle-shaped tumour cells, some with hyperchromatic nuclei, may be present. The tumour cells are arranged in irregular and moderately well defined masses and/or in strands of loosely connected cells in a lymphoid stroma. The tumour cells do not produce mucin. These cytological and histological features are fairly characteristic and when present in metastatic tumours, which are particularly common in the upper cervical lymph nodes, may enable a presumptive diagnosis of nasopharyngeal carcinoma to be made.

The term " *lymphoepithelial carcinoma* " [lymphoepithelioma] is used describe nonkeratinizing and undifferentiated nasopharyngeal carcinom in which numerous lymphocytes are found among the tumour cells. lymphoid elements in such tumours are not neoplastic. Lymphoepith carcinomas, like other undifferentiated carcinomas of the nasopha show ultrastructural evidence of squamous differentiation.

14. *Basal cell carcinoma :* A locally invasive, slowly spreading
     which rarely metastasises, arising in the epidermis or
     licles, and in which the peripheral cells usually simulate
     cells of the epidermis.

Basal cell carcinomas of the external ear exhibit the sam histological appearances as those arising in other sites.

15. *Ceruminous adenoma and adenocarcinoma* (Fig. 35–38): Tumours of ceruminous glands.

Ceruminous adenomas generally consist of bilayered glandular structures separated by variable stromal elements. They are not encapsulated. A biphasic pattern reminiscent of pleomorphic adenoma may be seen. Ceruminous tumours are similar to other apocrine gland tumours and show the same range of structural variation. The distinction between benign and malignant forms may be difficult on histological grounds. Metastases are exceedingly rare except in the case of adenoid cystic tumours arising from ceruminous glands (see para. 18).

16. *Adenocarcinoma* (Fig. 39–42): A malignant epithelial tumour of glandular structure.

These tumours may be trabecular, tubular, acinar, or papillary. Cystic forms may occur. Some adenocarcinomas, especially those with papillary structure, may arise from the surface epithelium as well as from glandular epithelium. Adenocarcinomas may occur in any part of the upper respiratory tract but are relatively more common in the ethmoid sinus and the upper part of the nasal cavity. They are distinguished from adenomas on the basis of anaplasia, infiltrative behaviour, and a high mitotic index. Well-differentiated adenocarcinomas may resemble adenomas closely but have a high frequency of local recurrence.

17. *Mucinous adenocarcinoma* (Fig. 43–44): An adenocarcinoma in which there is substantial mucus production by the tumour cells. The mucus may be intracellular or extracellular and is usually visible grossly.

The presence of signet ring cells and/or lakes of mucus is the characteristic histological feature of this type of adenocarcinoma. The structure is similar to that of mucinous adenocarcinomas of the gastro-intestinal tract.

18. *Adenoid cystic carcinoma* (Fig. 45–47): A malignant tumour having a characteristic cribriform structure. The tumour cells form small duct-like structures or larger masses with interspersed cystic spaces to give a cribriform or lace-like pattern.

This is the most commonly encountered malignant glandular tumour of the upper respiratory tract. The duct-like structures often contain eosinophilic PAS-positive material, and basophilic Alcian blue-positive mucoid material is found around the tumour masses and also within sharply defined round spaces among the tumour cells. Adenoid cystic carcinomas may show other cellular patterns in addition to the cribriform appearance. Tumours with a predominantly solid pattern are usually associated with a poorer prognosis. The tumour is typically infiltrative with a special tendency to grow along nerve sheaths. This tumour has been referred to as " cylindroma ".

19. *Mucoepidermoid carcinoma* (Fig. 48–50): A tumour characterized by the presence of squamous cells, mucus-secreting cells, and cells of intermediate type.

The ratio of squamous cells to mucous cells varies. Both mucous secretion and the presence of squamous cells should be demonstrable in any growth that is placed in this category. Furthermore, the mucoid and myxochondroid changes of the pleomorphic adenoma should not be present. The epidermoid component is usually present in the form of clumps or strands or as multi-layered masses between the mucous secreting epithelium. The squamous cells often have recognizable intercellular bridges, but well developed keratinization is uncommon. The intermediate type cells have hyperchromatic nuclei and scanty cytoplasm. Cells with clear cytoplasm may also be present. Mucus-filled cysts are seen frequently.

20. *Carcinoid tumour* (Fig. 51): A tumour of the diffuse endocrine system derived from Kulchitsky-type cells.

This neoplasm may show a trabecular pattern or a mixture of solid islands and trabeculae separated by fibrous stroma which is frequently hyalinized. The tumour cells are regular with uniform nuclei and granular eosinophilic or pale-staining cytoplasm. The peripheral layer of cells of each group tends to be orientated with the nuclei towards the centre of the group and the cytoplasm peripherally. Glandular lumina and rosette formation may also be seen with occasional palisading of cells, giving a neuroid appearance. Carcinoids of the upper respiratory tract are often negative with argentaffin techniques but the majority of cases show some argyrophilia, i.e., are silver-positive with a technique that uses an external reducing agent.

21. *Other malignant epithelial tumours*

Acinar cell adenocarcinoma, carcinoma in a pleomorphic adenoma [malignant mixed tumour], and *clear cell (glycogen-rich) adenocarcinoma* rarely occur in the upper respiratory tract. An intestinal type of adenocarcinoma has been described in the nasal cavity on the basis of resemblance to intestinal epithelium.

22. *Undifferentiated carcinoma* : A malignant epithelial tumour which does not show evidence of squamous or glandular differentiation or, in the nasal cavity and paranasal sinuses, any resemblance to " transitional " carcinoma.

Some of these tumours may exhibit a basaloid appearance due to palisading of cells at the periphery of the tumour masses.

SOFT TISSUE TUMOURS

23. *Soft tissue tumours*

These are generally classified and defined according to the scheme already published.[1] Only those more commonly encountered in the upper respiratory tract are listed here.

24. *Lipoma* (Fig. 52): A benign tumour made up of mature adipose tissue cells showing no evidence of cellular atypia.

The tumours are frequently intersected by bands of vascular fibrous tissue. Lipomas undergoing myxoid changes should not be confused with well-differentiated myxoid liposarcoma.

25. *Juvenile angiofibroma* (Fig. 53–54): A locally destructive tumour composed of fibrovascular tissue of varying maturity, arising in the wall of the nasopharynx.

The vascular elements of this neoplasm are randomly distributed and are a mixture of thick- and thin-walled vascular channels with interconnexions between the two. There may be focal thickening of the intima, forming so-called " cushions ". The thick-walled vessels may show irregular or incomplete layers of muscle of immature appearance. The stromal element consists of varying proportions of cellular and collagenous fibrous tissue. There may be numerous mast cells. Moderate cytological atypia and multinucleated cells are occasionally present. The proportion of vessels to stroma varies in individual cases. The neoplasm occurs almost exclusively in the nasopharynx of young males, particularly in the 10–25-year age group. Its occurrence in other parts of the upper respiratory tract is exceedingly rare.

---

[1] Enzinger, F. M., Lattes, R. & Torloni, H. (1969) *Histological typing of soft tissue tumours*, Geneva, World Health Organization (*International Histological Classification of Tumours*, No. 3).

26. *Haemangioma* (Fig. 55): A benign non-circumscribed lesion consisting of blood vessels of various types.

The nature of these lesions, i.e., whether they are hamartomatous or neoplastic, is not clear. In the upper respiratory tract they are usually of the capillary type. The condition must be distinguished from angiogranuloma (see para. 68), which occurs much more frequently in the upper respiratory tract.

27. *Haemangiopericytoma* (Fig. 56–57): A tumour characterized by the proliferation of round, oval, or spindle-shaped cells of rather uniform size surrounded by reticulin fibres and arranged about vascular spaces lined by a single layer of endothelial cells.

The perivascular arrangement of the tumour cells is well shown by reticulin staining. The tumour is uncommon and a clear separation from other well-vascularized mesenchymal tumours may be difficult. The clinical course is seldom predictable on the basis of histological findings.

28. *Leiomyoma :* A benign tumour of smooth muscle cells.

The tumour cells are spindle shaped and usually arranged in interlacing bundles. They are characterized by the presence of non-striated myofibrils within their cytoplasm.

29. *Rhabdomyoma* (Fig. 58): A benign tumour of immature striated muscle cells.

The tumour usually consists of large polygonal, frequently vacuolated (glycogen-containing) cells having abundant finely granular deeply eosinophilic cytoplasm. Cells with cross-striations are fairly common. The tumour is rare and the majority of cases have been observed in the upper neck region, the tongue, the pharyngeal wall, and the larynx.

30. *Granular cell tumour* (Fig. 59): A benign tumour made up of large, round, polygonal or elongated cells with finely granular eosinophilic cytoplasm.

The tumour is not encapsulated and the cells frequently extend into adjacent tissues. The cytoplasmic granules stain with PAS. Superficially located tumours are often accompanied by pseudo-epitheliomatous hyperplasia of the overlying squamous epithelium. This tumour is of debatable histogenesis. It has been referred to as " granular cell myoblastoma " but recent evidence does not support a myoblastic origin.

31. *Neurofibroma* (Fig. 60): A benign tumour consisting of a mixture of Schwann cells and fibroblasts in a collagenous or oedematous matrix.

The tumour cells are spindle shaped, have elongated nuclei, and are arranged in streams or twisted bundles. Axons can frequently be demonstrated in the tumour. In contrast to neurilemmomas (see para. 32), these tumours are not well demarcated. Plexiform neurofibromas are the result of growth within and about a preformed nerve, giving the nerve trunk a tortuous, thickened, and plexiform appearance. Malignant transformation of neurofibromas may occur. Neurofibromas of the upper respiratory tract occur in an isolated form or as part of von Recklinghausen's disease (neurofibromatosis).

32. *Neurilemmoma* [schwannoma] (Fig. 61): A benign tumour of Schwann cells which is usually well demarcated or encapsulated.

Characteristically, an Antoni type A pattern with regimentation of the nuclei in twisted rows or palisades (Verocay bodies) and an Antoni type B pattern with loosely arranged cells within a wide-meshed microcystic fibrillar stroma may be recognized. Perivascular hyalinization is common. Axons are not demonstrable within the tumour. There is no tendency for malignant transformation to occur. The tumours are often highly vascular and may present secondary features such as haemorrhage, thrombosis, phagocytosis of lipid and haemosiderin, and cystic changes. There may be aggregates of foam cells and areas with cellular pleomorphism.

33. *Myxoma* (Fig. 62): A benign tumour of unknown histogenesis characterized by rather small inconspicuous spindle or stellate cells within a myxoid matrix.

The matrix is composed of abundant mucoid material, chiefly hyaluronic acid, a loose meshwork of reticulin, and collagen fibrils. The lesion is poorly vascularized. The tumours show locally infiltrative growth and tend to recur. Fat stains are helpful in distinguishing this condition from myxoid liposarcoma.

34. *Fibroxanthoma* [fibrous histiocytoma] (Fig. 63): A benign, unencapsulated growth made up of histiocytes and collagen-producing fibroblast-like cells which may be arranged in a storiform pattern. Frequently, the growth contains lipid-carrying macrophages—foam cells and Touton-type giant cells—and inflammatory cells. It may have a prominent vascular component.

35. *Paraganglioma* [chemodectoma] (Fig. 64–67): A tumour of a chemoreceptor organ or extra-adrenal paraganglia.

These tumours consist of a dense capillary network enclosing aggregations of tumour cells (" Zellballen "). The vascular or the parenchymal elements may predominate in the histological picture and, on this basis, adenoma-like and angioma-like types have been described in addition to the typical pattern. The chief tumour cell has epithelioid features with abundant finely granular cytoplasm with a moth-eaten appearance, and a round or oval vesicular nucleus. Spindle-shaped cells may also be present. The tumour cells are typically arranged in alveolar compartments that are best demonstrated with a reticulin stain. Nuclear hyperchromatism and pleomorphism do not provide a reliable basis for the distinction between benign and malignant paraganglioma. Tumours of the glomus jugulare are not encapsulated. Stromal haemosiderin deposits and a chronic inflammatory reaction may be present.

36. *Fibrosarcoma* : A malignant tumour composed of predominantly spindle shaped cells producing reticulin and occasionally collagen and showing no evidence of other forms of cellular differentiation.

The histological picture consists of interlacing cellular fascicles often forming a herringbone pattern. There is a close relationship between cells and reticulin fibres. The degree of differentiation is of prognostic significance. Well-differentiated tumours consist of bundles of uniform spindle cells in a collagenous matrix. Mitoses are few. Poorly differentiated tumours are richly cellular with minimal intercellular ground substance. They may exhibit marked cellular pleomorphism and numerous mitoses.

37. *Rhabdomyosarcoma* (Fig. 68–74): A malignant tumour of rhabdomyoblasts and primitive mesenchymal tissue.

This tumour is classified into *embryonal, alveolar,* and *pleomorphic* types according to the *predominant* pattern. The type occurring most frequently in the upper respiratory tract is the embryonal. In this variety the tumour cells are relatively small and have varying amounts of eosinophilic cytoplasm in which cross-striations may be demonstrated. The demonstration of cross-striations is not essential for the diagnosis of rhabdomyosarcoma. The stroma is oedematous and myxoid. Rhabdomyosarcomas are highly malignant tumours and in the upper respiratory tract and the middle ear are usually encountered in the first decade of life. The term " sarcoma botryoides " is applied clinically to submucosal tumours which form polypoid grape-like structures. Such lesions generally consist of an oedematous or myxoid matrix with scanty tumour cells except for a richly cellular zone close to the epithelial surface.

38. *Angiosarcoma* (Fig. 75): A malignant neoplasm characterized by the formation of irregular anastomosing vascular channels lined by anaplastic endothelial cells which may pile up to form tufts.

39. *Kaposi's sarcoma :* A malignant tumour composed of irregular vascular channels and spaces formed and surrounded by slender spindle shaped cells with prominent deeply staining nuclei superficially resembling leiomyoblasts.

In the upper respiratory tract, the lesions occur most frequently in the larynx, and only as part of a systemic disease. The presence of extravasations of erythrocytes and of haemosiderin pigment are common. There is also a nonspecific inflammatory infiltrate.

40. *Neurogenic sarcoma* [neurofibrosarcoma and malignant schwannoma] (Fig. 76): A malignant tumour consisting of spindle shaped cells of neurogenic origin.

The tumour is usually densely cellular and contains frequent mitoses. Cellular pleomorphism and the presence of collagen fibres are characteristic features. Nuclear palisading as well as arrangement of the cells in groups, nests, cords, or whorls are helpful in differential diagnosis. The tumour is frequently related to a nerve trunk. The distinction between a neurofibrosarcoma and malignant schwannoma is based on the identification of a remnant of the corresponding benign tumour. Origin in a pre-existing neurofibroma is frequent but origin in a neurilemmoma is exceedingly rare.

41. *Malignant fibroxanthoma* [malignant fibrous histiocytoma] (Fig. 77–78): This is the malignant counterpart of the fibroxanthoma (see para. 34), from which it is distinguished by higher mitotic activity, pleomorphism, and infiltrative behaviour.

TUMOURS OF BONE AND CARTILAGE

42. *Tumours of bone and cartilage*

These are classified and defined according to the scheme already published.[1]

Almost any tumour or tumour-like lesion of bone or cartilage may involve the upper respiratory tract. Particular problems are encountered

---

[1] Schajowicz, F., Ackerman, L. V., Sissons, H. A., Sobin, L. H. & Torloni, H. (1972) *Histological typing of bone tumours*, Geneva, World Health Organization (*International Histological Classification of Tumours*, No. 6).

when these grow into the paranasal sinuses. The most common benign tumours are osteoma and chondroma. Malignant tumours are rare. The most frequent tumour-like lesions are fibrous dysplasia and giant cell " reparative " granuloma.

43. *Chondroma* (Fig. 79): A benign tumour characterized by the formation of mature cartilage, and lacking the high cellularity, pleomorphism, large binucleated cells, and mitoses seen in chondrosarcoma.

44. *Osteoma* (Fig. 80): A benign slow-growing lesion consisting of well-differentiated mature bone tissue with a predominantly lamellar structure.

These lesions are regarded by some as hamartomas rather than true neoplasms. Such lesions in the external auditory meatus have been termed exostoses. Osteomas may grow into the paranasal sinuses, mainly the frontal and ethmoidal sinuses, as bony masses of varying density.

45. *Ossifying fibroma* (Fig. 81): A benign but locally aggressive fibro-osseous lesion consisting of spindle-shaped fibroblastic cells usually arranged in a whorled pattern and containing small islands and spicules of metaplastic woven bone and mineralized masses.

The lesion is found most frequently in the maxilla of young subjects and may appear encapsulated. Mitosis may be present. The bony spicules may rarely show a lamellar structure peripherally and are frequently rimmed by osteoblasts. The lesion may be difficult to distinguish from fibrous dysplasia (see para. 75).

46. *Chondrosarcoma* (Fig. 82): A malignant tumour characterized by the formation of cartilage, but not of bone, by the tumour cells.

The tumour is distinguished from chondroma by the presence of more cellular and pleomorphic tumour tissue, and clusters of plump cells with large or double nuclei. Mitotic cells are infrequent. Chondrosarcomas frequently show areas of calcification and endochondral ossification, but neither bone nor osteoid is formed by the tumour cells.

47. *Osteosarcoma* (Fig. 83): A malignant tumour characterized by the direct formation of bone or osteoid tissue by the tumour cells.

Osteosarcomas vary in the amount of tumour bone or osteoid present and in the pleomorphism of the tumour cells. The tumour cells may produce cartilage and there may be areas where the tumour cells are undifferentiated and resemble fibrosarcoma. Direct osteoid production by the tumour cells distinguishes the condition from chondrosarcoma, in which endochondral ossification may occur (see para. 46).

TUMOURS OF LYMPHOID AND HAEMATOPOIETIC TISSUES

48. *Malignant lymphomas* (Fig. 84–88)

Any of the types of malignant lymphoma may arise as a primary tumour in the upper respiratory tract. Primary Hodgkin's disease, however, is exceedingly rare in this area. These tumours are described in detail elsewhere.[1] Lymphomas of the upper respiratory tract may exhibit necrotic and inflammatory changes that may obscure the malignant lymphoreticular elements. Such tumours may be difficult to distinguish from lethal midline granuloma (see para. 82).

49. *Plasmacytoma* (Fig. 88): A malignant tumour formed exclusively of plasma cells in varying stages of maturation.

The upper respiratory tract is the most frequent site of extramedullary plasmacytoma. While presenting in the upper respiratory tract, such tumours may later prove to be part of a systemic disease. The tumour cells vary from normal-looking plasma cells with the characteristic eccentric nuclei and amphophilic cytoplasm to less mature cells which are more pleomorphic and have larger and more centrally placed nuclei. Binuclear forms may be present. The tumour cells are arranged in sheets and there is a delicate vascular stroma. Amyloid may be present. Inflammatory cells are not present except near ulcerated surfaces. The condition should be distinguished from plasma cell granuloma (see para. 80).

MISCELLANEOUS TUMOURS

50. *Teratoma* (Fig. 89–90): A tumour composed of multiple tissues that are foreign to their sites of occurrence and are typically derived from more than one germ layer.

Teratomas are encountered most commonly in childhood. They may be divided into *solid* and *cystic* forms. The *dermoid cyst* is composed of one or more cysts lined by epidermis with skin appendages.

---

[1] Mathé, G., Rappaport, H., O'Conor, G. T. & Torloni, H. (1976) *Histological and cytological typing of neoplastic diseases of haematopoietic and lymphoid tissues*, Geneva, World Health Organization (*International Histological Classification of Tumours*, No. 14).

In general, benign and malignant teratomas are distinguished on the basis of anaplasia and invasive growth. However, benign teratomas in infancy may contain immature developing tissues, mainly of neurogenic origin.

51. *Pituitary adenoma* (Fig. 91–92): A benign tumour composed of anterior pituitary type cells.

The tumour cells are typically of the chromophobe variety and may be arranged in sheets, columns, or nests, which are separated by thin-walled vascular channels or connective tissue trabeculae. The tumour is rare and represents a downward extension from a suprasellar neoplasm more often than origin from a pharyngeal pituitary in the nasopharynx.

52. *Meningioma* (Fig. 93–94): A tumour of meningothelial cells.

The tumour cells are characteristically spindle-shaped and arranged in concentric onion-skin-like whorls around small blood vessels, with or without the formation of psammoma bodies. Nests and sheets of polygonal cells may also be present. The tumour may arise primarily in the nasal cavity and sinuses or may represent a local extension from an intracranial tumour.

53. *Odontogenic tumours* (Fig. 95–96):

A variety of odontogenic tumours may extend into the nasal cavities. These tumours, which are illustrated and described in detail elsewhere,[1] may also occur as primary tumours in the maxillary antrum.

Cementifying fibroma, in which small basophilic masses of calcified cementum-like tissues are found in a cellular fibroblastic stroma, may occasionally present features resembling ossifying fibroma (see para. 45).

54. *Melanotic neuroectodermal tumour* [melanotic progonoma] (Fig. 97–98): A rare benign tumour, probably of neural crest derivation, that occurs mostly in the maxilla of young infants.

The tumour consists of tubules or spaces separated by prominent fibrous tissue stroma. The spaces are generally lined by cuboidal epithelial cells with pale nuclei and fairly abundant cytoplasm in which melanin pigment is frequently identified. Smaller cells with hyperchromatic nuclei and scanty cytoplasm are frequently found within these spaces. The tumour is usually nonencapsulated and may be locally aggressive but has a benign clinical course.

---

[1] Pindborg, J. J., Kramer, I. R. H. & Torloni, H. (1971) *Histological typing of odontogenic tumours, jaw cysts, and allied lesions*, Geneva, World Health Organization (*International Histological Classification of Tumours*, No. 5).

55. *Malignant melanoma* (Fig. 99): A malignant neoplasm of melano-
cytes.

Malignant melanomas of the upper respiratory tract exhibit the full
range of structure found in those arising in the skin, but have a poorer prognosis than the cutaneous forms.

56. *Olfactory neurogenic [esthesioneurogenic] tumours* (Fig. 100–105):
A malignant neoplasm considered to be of olfactory neural
membrane origin and composed of clusters or masses of neurogenic cells with diffusely distributed nuclear chromatin and a
neurofibrillar matrix.

The tumours exhibit a distinctive lobular or fascicular architecture. Three
histological varieties have been recognized: *Esthesioneurocytoma* (Fig. 100–
103)—The cells in this type have uniform, small nuclei and a fairly prominent neurofibrillar matrix. Mitoses are not found. Foci of calcification and
pseudorosettes are frequently present. *Esthesioneuroepithelioma* (Fig. 104)
—The cells in this type exhibit increased anaplasia. True rosettes are a
distinctive feature. *Esthesioneuroblastoma* (Fig. 105)—The cells in this type
exhibit pleomorphism and the neurofibrillar matrix is scarce. Pseudorosettes
may be identified.

57. *Chordoma* (Fig. 106): A tumour, presumed to be of notochordal
origin, characterized by lobulated masses and cords of pleomorphic vacuolated cells and mucoid intercellular material.

The most characteristic type of tumour cell is a voluminous polyhedral
cell with a vacuolated cytoplasm (physaliphorous cells). The vacuolated
cells contain glycogen. Nonvacuolated fusiform and stellate cells also occur.
The tumour is frequently intersected by fibrous trabeculae. This is a rare
neoplasm that occurs mainly in relation to the axial skeleton, particularly
in the spheno-occipital and sacral regions. The tumour is slow-growing and
locally infiltrative and recurs after removal; metastases are rare. It should
be distinguished from chondrosarcoma and mucin-secreting carcinoma.

58. *Craniopharyngioma* (Fig. 107–108): A tumour of the vestigial
remnants of the craniopharyngeal duct (Rathke's pouch).

The neoplasm consists of irregular masses and thick branching cords of
stratified epithelium separated by a loose connective tissue matrix. The cells
in the inner portions of the epithelial masses appear stellate. The columnar
or basal epithelial cells adjoining the stroma show palisading reminiscent

of ameloblastoma. Intercellular oedema is usually present and may progress to cyst formation. Cysts may also develop from stromal degeneration. Tubular and/or glandular structures may be present. Keratinization is often prominent and there may be foci of calcification and ossification. Craniopharyngiomas can be predominantly cystic or solid. They may cause localized pressure necrosis of tissues and may be locally invasive.

TUMOUR-LIKE LESIONS

59. *Pseudoepitheliomatous hyperplasia* (Fig. 109): An irregular over-growth of squamous epithelium with tumour-like extensions into the stroma.

The epithelium is well differentiated and does not exhibit any cytological evidence of malignancy. The epithelial extensions may appear separated from the surface and should not be mistaken for invasion. This reaction is an exaggerated epithelial response in the process of repair and may be observed in chronic inflammatory and ulcerative lesions and with granular cell tumours.

60. *Keratosis obturans :* A form of hyperkeratosis in which there is accumulation of large amounts of desquamated keratin in the external auditory canal, which may lead to pressure atrophy of bone.

61. *Epidermoid " cholesteatoma "* (Fig. 110): A cyst-like lesion of the middle ear cleft lined by keratinizing squamous epithelium and filled with laminated masses of keratin.

The lesion generally occurs as a complication of otitis media and may be associated with a chronic inflammatory reaction. Cholesterol deposits are occasionally present. The accumulation of keratin may cause pressure necrosis of surrounding bony structures.

62. *Epithelial abnormalities.*

Certain terms—leukoplakia, pachydermia—are used to describe epithelial abnormalities clinically. Their use for histological diagnosis is not justified. The term 'leukoplakia' should be restricted to a clinical description of a white patch on the mucosal surface.

63. *Keratosis/epithelial hyperplasia of the larynx* [keratosis without atypia] (Fig. 111–112): Lesions in which there is thickening of the squamous epithelium without cellular atypia. Keratosis refers to the presence of keratin or parakeratin; a granular layer is often evident. Epithelial hyperplasia (acanthosis) refers to an increase in the number of prickle cell layers. These abnormalities frequently co-exist.

64. *Dysplasia* [keratosis with atypia] (Fig. 113): A lesion in which part of the thickness of the epithelium reveals varying degrees of cellular atypia and/or loss of normal stratification short of carcinoma in situ. Keratotic changes may be seen. Some degree of surface maturation is present. Three grades of dysplasia— mild, moderate, and severe—are commonly described.

65. *Oncocytic metaplasia and hyperplasia* [oncocytosis] (Fig. 114): A proliferative lesion comprising large glandular cells with abundant granular eosinophilic cytoplasm, typically arranged in a bilayered pattern.

This change may affect parts, or the whole, of glandular units. When extensive or nodular, this lesion may be difficult to distinguish from oxyphilic adenoma (see para. 5).

66. *Cysts* (Fig. 115–116).

Two types of cysts may be found in the upper respiratory tract. *Retention* cysts are brought about by obstruction of ducts. *Developmental* cysts arise from ectopic epithelial tissues or from vestigial remnants, e.g., branchial cleft and Rathke's pouch elements. These cysts may be lined by a variety of epithelia and may contain keratin or cholesterol.

67. *Mucocele*

This is a retention phenomenon of the paranasal sinuses which produces a cystic cavity lined by sinus epithelium. The contents are generally mucinous but may be haemorrhagic or purulent. Pressure destruction of adjacent bony walls can occur.

68. *Angiogranuloma* [" haemangioma " of granulation tissue type, granuloma pyogenicum] (Fig. 117–120): A rapidly growing, often ulcerated lesion with the appearance of richly vascular granulation tissue.

Histological differentiation between benign vascular tumours and angiogranuloma can be difficult, and, at times, impossible. The topography of angiogranuloma is based on the development and maturation of granulation tissue in which a proliferating capillary bed is supplied by branches of small muscular arteries. The vascular loop is completed by small post-capillary venules. In favourably oriented sections this developmental sequence is seen as a lobular pattern of endothelial and fibroblastic proliferation related to the dichotomously branching feeder artery. In contrast, the topography of a true vascular neoplasm presents a randomly distributed pattern of capillary channels without a consistent relationship to feeder vessels; cavernous channels may be present and, at times, are seen directly beneath the overlying epithelium. Diagnostic difficulties arise from secondary inflammation in haemangiomas and unfavourable orientation of angiogranuloma in biopsy material.

69. *Intubation granuloma/" contact " ulcer* (Fig. 121): A tumour-like mass of granulation tissue or ulcerative lesion resulting from laryngeal trauma/intubation.

The lesion is invariably found on the vocal processes of the arytenoid cartilages. It may be histologically similar to angiogranuloma and may be accompanied by pseudoepitheliomatous hyperplasia.

70. *Nasal polyp* (Fig. 122–123): A projection of oedematous nasal mucosa covered by respiratory epithelium with varying numbers of goblet cells.

Polyps are common lesions in the nasal cavity and paranasal sinuses; they may also present through the choana (antro-choanal polyps). The surface epithelium may show foci of ulceration and varying degrees of squamous metaplasia. The basement membrane is often thickened and hyalinized. The oedematous stroma may show pseudocysts and is infiltrated by lymphocytes, plasma cells, eosinophils, and mast cells; in the so-called allergic type, eosinophils predominate. Accumulations of atypical stromal cells may be seen.

71. *Vocal cord polyp* (Fig. 124–126): A polypoid or nodular lesion of the vocal cord.

The lesion is covered by stratified squamous epithelium and may exhibit a variety of changes in the stroma. These include oedema, fibrosis, increased vascularity and haemorrhage, hyaline changes, and myxoid changes. Vocal cord polyps may be divided into *fibrous, vascular, hyalinized,* and *myxoid* polyps on the basis of these stromal changes.

72. *Otic [aural] polyp* (Fig. 127): A polypoid lesion in the auditory meatus or middle ear, consisting of inflammatory granulation tissue covered by columnar or squamous epithelium.

This lesion frequently originates in the middle ear and projects into the auditory meatus through a perforated tympanic membrane. Chronic inflammatory changes, often associated with foreign body reaction to keratin or cholesterol, are present. Gland-like structures may be present. The surface epithelium may be ulcerated.

73. *Keloid* (Fig. 128): A superficial nodular parvicellular growth formed by fibrocytic and/or fibroblastic cells lying between well-defined interlacing broad bands of homogeneous acidophilic collagen. The lesion usually follows some form of injury and has a tendency to recur.

74. *Fibromatosis* (Fig. 129): A locally aggressive tumour-like fibroblastic growth.

The lesion has a strong tendency to local recurrence and aggressive infiltrating growth. It varies in cellularity and may be distinguished from well-differentiated fibrosarcoma by its uniform growth pattern, abundance of collagen, paucity of mitotic figures, and lack of metastasis. The lesion is of unknown pathogenesis.

75. *Fibrous dysplasia* (Fig. 130): A self-limiting, presumably developmental, non-encapsulated lesion showing replacement of normal bone by fibrous connective tissue of varying cellularity and containing islands of trabecular or immature nonlamellar metaplastic bone.

Cellular fibrous tissue predominates in the early lesions and the amount of bone increases with the stage of development of the lesion. Osteoblastic rimming is absent or inconspicuous. Cystic changes and osteoclasts may be present. The lesion is usually located in the maxilla of young subjects; in the maxilla the lesion is usually monostotic and may be difficult to distinguish from ossifying fibroma (see para. 45).

76. *Giant cell "reparative" granuloma* (Fig. 131): An intraosseous lesion consisting of cellular fibrous tissue containing foci of haemorrhage and aggregations of multinucleated giant cells.

The multinucleated giant cells exhibit benign cytological features and are usually found in relation to capillaries and foci of haemorrhage. Trabeculae of woven bone may be formed within septa of more mature fibrous tissue that may traverse the lesion. The lesion occurs more frequently in children and young adults. The benign fibroblastic appearance of the stromal cells serves to distinguish the lesion from true giant cell tumours, which occur only rarely in the jaws. The brown tumour of hyperparathyroidism is histologically indistinguishable from giant cell " reparative " granuloma.

77. *Amyloid deposits* (Fig. 132):

Localized amyloid deposits may cause tumour-like lesions in the upper respiratory tract. The majority of these are found in the larynx but do not involve the true vocal cord. The appearance and staining characteristics of amyloid in this location are similar to those in other parts of the body. A prominent foreign body giant cell reaction may be seen.

78. *Infective granulomas* (Fig. 133–136).

A variety of infections may give rise to tumour-like lesions in the upper respiratory tract. These include *rhinoscleroma, rhinosporidiosis, tuberculosis, leishmaniasis,* and *histoplasmosis.*

The nodular tumour-like masses in *rhinoscleroma* (Fig. 133) are found mainly in the nasal cavity and less often in other parts of the upper respiratory tract. They are characterized by heavy infiltration by plasma cells, lymphocytes, and large macrophages with abundant clear or vacuolated cytoplasm (Mikulicz cells) in which Gram-negative bacilli (*Klebsiella rhinoscleromatis*) may be identified. There are numerous Russel bodies. In *rhinosporidiosis* (Fig. 134), caused by the endosporulating fungus *Rhinosporidium seeberi,* polypoid lesions occur principally in the nasal cavity and rarely in the larynx. The lesions are characterized by the presence of thick-walled sporangia measuring 50–350 microns in diameter and containing numerous spores. They are associated with a heavy chronic inflammatory reaction with occasional foci of suppuration and foreign body giant cell reaction. The lesions in *tuberculosis* (Fig. 135) are found more frequently in the larynx and are often ulcerated. The lesions in *leishmaniasis* and *histoplasmosis* (Fig. 136) are associated with heavy infiltration by inflammatory cells in the early stages and with tuberculoid granulomas and fibrosis in the late stages. The lesions in leishmaniasis occur more commonly in the nasal cavity and are markedly destructive. The protozoan parasite causing nasal leishmaniasis (*Leishmania braziliensis*) and the yeast-like fungus causing histoplasmosis (*Histoplasma capsulatum*) are usually found in large numbers within macrophages in the respective lesions.

79. *Cholesterol granuloma* (Fig. 137): A granulomatous lesion containing cholesterol crystals associated with a foreign body giant cell reaction and chronic inflammatory changes.

This lesion is a sequel to infection of the middle ear cleft or haemorrhage into the tympanic cavity. Inflammation may lead to a tumorous submucosal collection of cholesterol and inflammatory debris. It may be associated with epidermoid cholesteatoma (see para. 61).

80. *Plasma cell granuloma :* A tumour-like lesion in which plasma cells predominate.

The lesion is not associated with major abnormalities of protein metabolism or evidence of bone marrow involvement. It is distinguished from plasmacytoma (see para. 49) by the maturity of the plasma cells and admixture with chronic inflammatory cells. Focal accumulations of amyloid may be present.

81. *Benign lymphoid hyperplasia* [" adenoids "] (Fig. 138): A tumour-like lesion composed of hyperplastic lymphoid tissue. Lymphoid follicles with germinal centres are present. There may be inflammatory changes.

82. *Lethal midline granuloma* [Stewart's granuloma, " malignant " granuloma] (Fig. 139–141).

A progressively destructive non-tuberculoid granulomatous lesion occurring in the nasal cavity, paranasal sinuses, or palate. This lesion is pleomorphocellular and consists mainly of lymphocytes and histiocytes admixed with varying proportions of plasma cells and neutrophils. Histiocytes with abnormal nuclei and immature lymphoid cells are frequently present and such cases, which may be difficult to distinguish histologically from malignant lymphomas (see para. 48), have been referred to as " lethal midline reticulosis " or " pleomorphic reticulosis ".

The lesion is frequently associated with extensive necrosis. There may be thrombosis of small vessels, but vasculitis and giant cells are generally absent. These features serve to distinguish the lesions from Wegener's granulomatosis (see para. 83). A small proportion of cases, however, may show vasculitis and occasional giant cells.

Lethal midline granuloma may involve contiguous structures, with necrosis of bone and orbital tissues and ulceration of the face, but there is generally no systemic involvement. The clinical and histological features have suggested a locally aggressive lympho-proliferative disorder that may possibly represent an abnormal hypersensitivity reaction. Since some of these lesions have been shown to terminate with systemic involvement, it has also been suggested that the lesion may be related to malignant lymphomas (see para. 48). The nosology of the lesion is debatable.

83. *Wegener's granulomatosis* (Fig. 142–143).

An immunologically mediated inflammatory disease in which granulomatous lesions in the upper respiratory tract occur in association with necrotizing granulomatous vasculitis in the lungs, glomerulitis, and disseminated small-vessel vasculitis. The lesions in the respiratory tract occur mainly in the nasal cavity and paranasal sinuses. The inflammatory cells do not exhibit cytological atypia. Giant cells and vasculitis are present. Lesions localized to the upper respiratory tract without systemic manifestations may rarely occur.

84. *Histiocytosis X* (Fig. 144): A group of diseases of obscure nature in which there are infiltrations by mature histiocytes and varying proportions of eosinophils, foamy histiocytes, and giant cells.

The clinico-pathological entities which comprise this group are eosinophilic granuloma, Hand-Schüller-Christian disease, and Letterer-Siwe disease. *Eosinophilic granuloma* is a localized form of histiocytosis found mostly in young adults. The lesions are usually limited to a single bone or organ and are characterized by a predominance of eosinophils. This disease has a good prognosis. *Hand-Schüller-Christian disease* is a chronic disseminated form of histiocytosis occurring mainly in children. The lesions tend to involve multiple bones and possibly other tissues. The cellular infiltrate comprises varying proportions of mature histiocytes, eosinophils, foam cells, and giant cells; neutrophils, lymphocytes, and plasma cells may also be present and the lesions may undergo fibrosis. The disease has a prolonged course. *Letterer-Siwe disease* is an acute systemic form of histiocytosis with prominent visceral and cutaneous involvement, occurring mainly in infants. The lesions are characterized by a predominance of histiocytes. The disease is usually rapidly fatal. It is distinguished from malignant histiocytosis by the absence of cytological evidence of malignancy.

85. *Nasal glial heterotopia* [nasal " glioma "] (Fig. 145–146): A tumour-like mass of mature glial tissue occurring intranasally in the upper part of the nasal cavity and/or at the base of the nose.

The glial tissue may include protoplasmic and gemistocytic astrocytes simulating nerve cells but there are no neurons; the formerly used synonym " ganglioglioma " is therefore a misnomer.

86. *Meningocele/meningoencephalocele :* An extracranial extrusion or herniation of the meninges or of meninges with brain tissue.

In the upper respiratory tract, these lesions may occur in the nasofrontal region and the nasal cavity. The presence of neurons and/or of a fluid-filled sac distinguishes this lesion from nasal glial heterotopias (see para. 85).

87. *Tracheopathia osteochondroplastica* (Fig. 147): A tumour-like lesion of the trachea, characterized by the formation of multiple sub-mucosal nodules composed of calcified and ossified cartilage.

88. *Chondrodermatitis nodularis chronica helicis* (Fig. 148–149): A necro-tizing chronic inflammatory process involving the perichondrial soft tissues and cartilage of the external ear.

The surface epithelium is often ulcerated and may show pseudo-epithelio-matous hyperplasia and hyperkeratosis. There are inflammatory changes and fibrinoid necrosis in the stroma. Although injury has been implicated, the etiology is obscure.

89. *Tympanosclerosis* (Fig. 150): A lesion characterized by dense hyalinized fibrous tissue covering the walls of the tympanic cavity and ossicles, frequently associated with patchy or diffuse calcifica-tion and bone formation.

INDEX

Unless otherwise stated, all the preparations shown in the photomicrographs reproduced on the following pages were stained with haematoxylin-eosin.

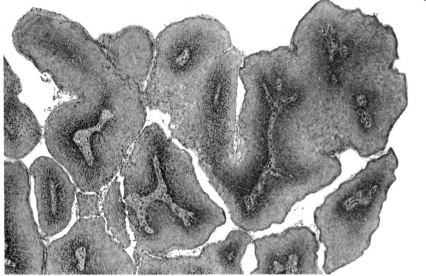

× 65

Fig. 1. Squamous cell papilloma, nasal cavity
Exophytic tumour of well-differentiated stratified squamous epithelium

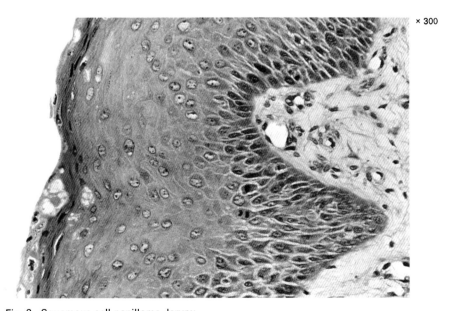

× 300

Fig. 2. Squamous cell papilloma, larynx
Well-differentiated, keratinizing, stratified squamous epithelium. Occasional mitoses

× 40

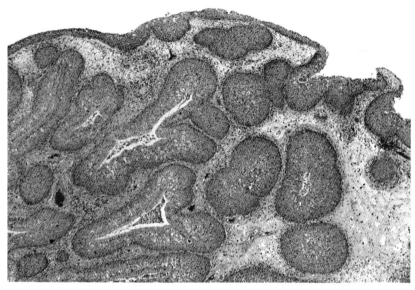

Fig. 3. '' Transitional '' papilloma, nasal cavity
Inverted type. Infolded tumour of nasal epithelium

× 65

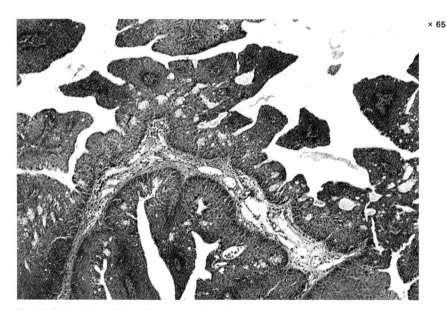

Fig. 4. '' Transitional '' papilloma, nasal cavity
Exophytic type. Stromal stalks lined by stratified and pseudostratified nasal epithelium

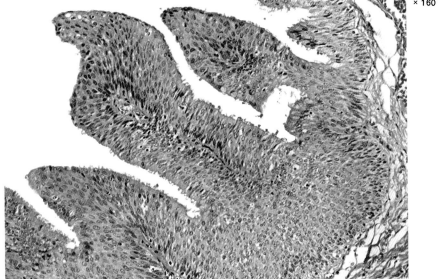

Fig. 5. '' Transitional '' papilloma, nasal cavity
Exophytic type. Outward growth of nasal respiratory epithelium

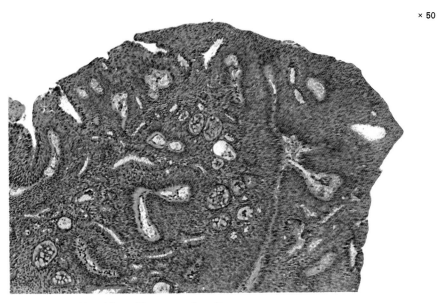

Fig. 6. '' Transitional '' papilloma, nasal cavity
Stratified and pseudostratified epithelium with mucus cells and mucus-filled microcysts.
Mucicarmine

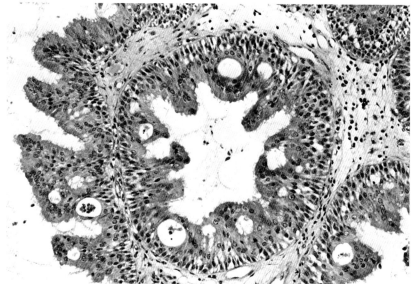

× 160

Fig. 7. '' Transitional '' papilloma, nasal cavity
Columnar cell type. Pseudostratified respiratory epithelium containing mucus-filled microcysts

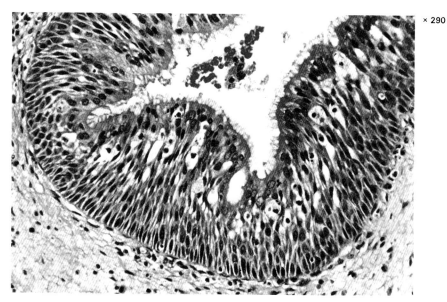

× 290

Fig. 8. '' Transitional '' papilloma, nasal cavity
Columnar cell type. Pseudostratified ciliated respiratory epithelium

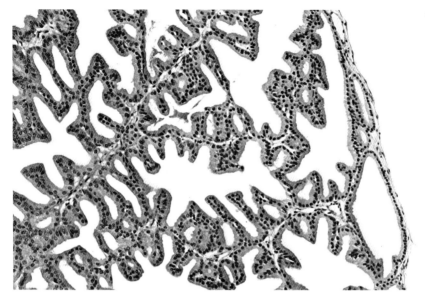

× 160

Fig. 9. Adenoma, nasal cavity
Glandular papillary structure

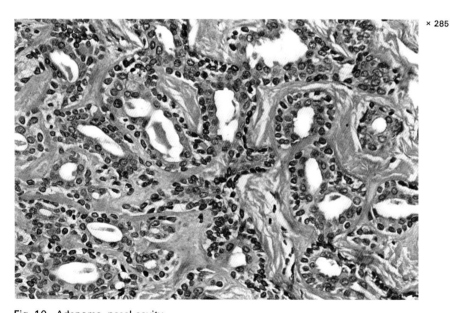

× 285

Fig. 10. Adenoma, nasal cavity
Tubular structure. Bilayered epithelium

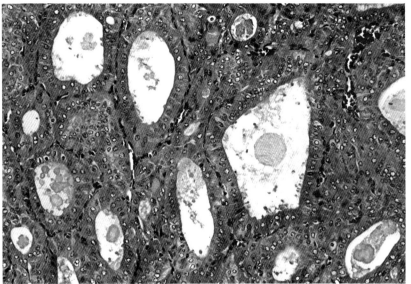

× 160

Fig. 11. Oxyphilic adenoma, nasal cavity
Glandular tumour composed of columnar cells with eosinophilic cytoplasm

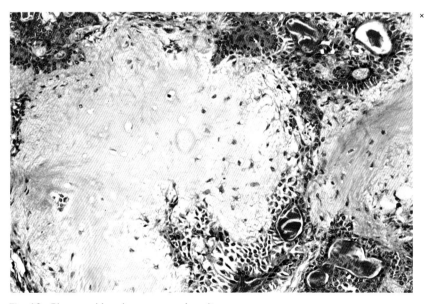

× 170

Fig. 12. Pleomorphic adenoma, nasal cavity
Epithelial and chondroid elements

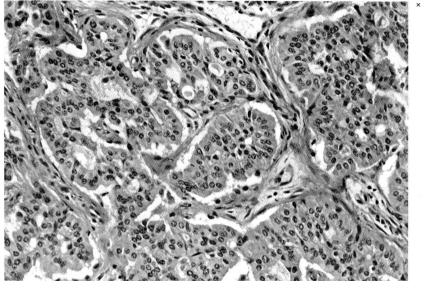

Fig 13. Adenoma of the middle ear
Glandular pattern

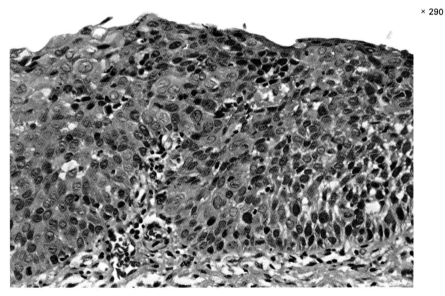

Fig. 14. Carcinoma in situ, larynx

× 350

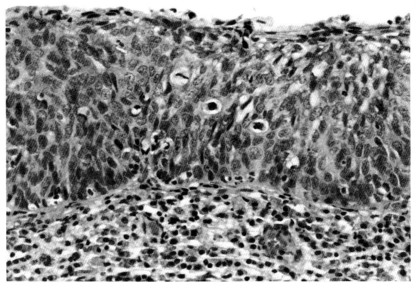

Fig. 15. Carcinoma in situ, larynx

× 250

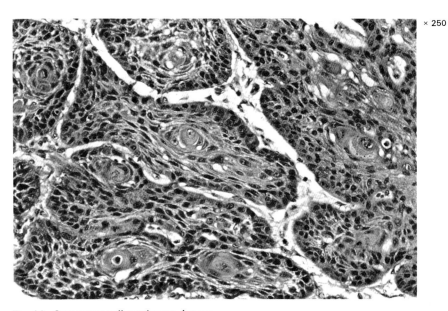

Fig. 16. Squamous cell carcinoma, larynx
Well differentiated. Infiltrating nests of squamous epithelium with keratinization and intercellular bridges

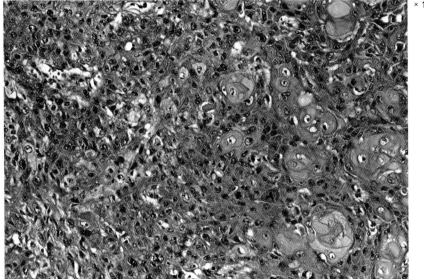

× 160

Fig. 17. Squamous cell carcinoma, larynx
Moderately differentiated and poorly differentiated areas

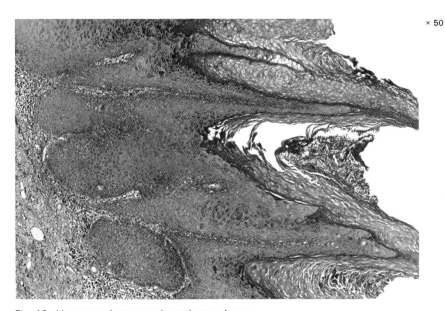

× 50

Fig. 18. Verrucous (squamous) carcinoma, larynx
Vertical folds of well-differentiated squamous epithelium capped by thick keratotic layer

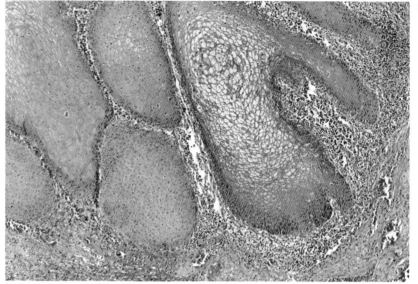

× 65

Fig. 19. Verrucous (squamous) carcinoma, larynx
Deep portion of tumour showing bulbous extensions into stroma. Same case as Fig. 18

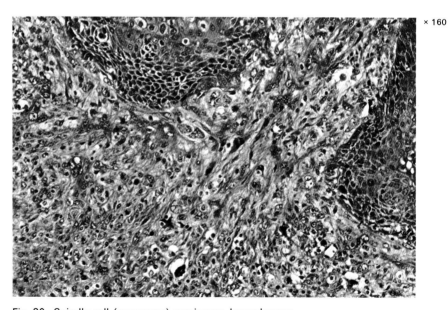

× 160

Fig. 20. Spindle cell (squamous) carcinoma, hypopharynx
Biphasic appearance. Well-differentiated squamous component and a pleomorphic spindle cell component

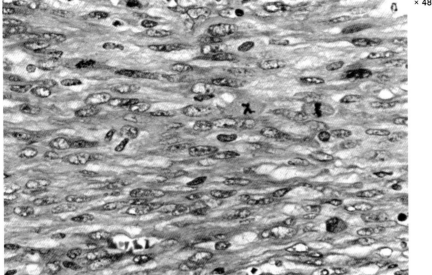

×480

Fig. 21. Spindle cell (squamous) carcinoma, larynx
Squamous cell carcinoma with pseudosarcomatous, spindle-celled structure

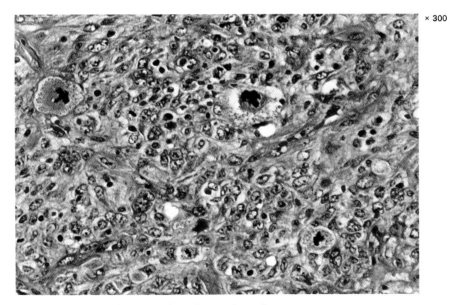

×300

Fig. 22. Spindle cell (squamous) carcinoma, hypopharynx
Cellular pleomorphism. Same case as Fig. 20

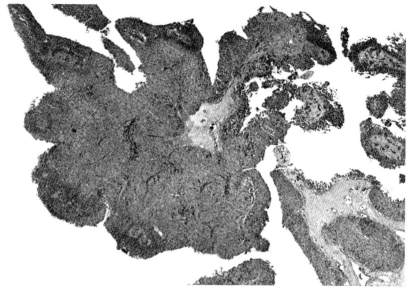

× 40

Fig. 23. " Transitional " carcinoma, nasal cavity
Exophytic tumour of nonkeratinizing epithelium

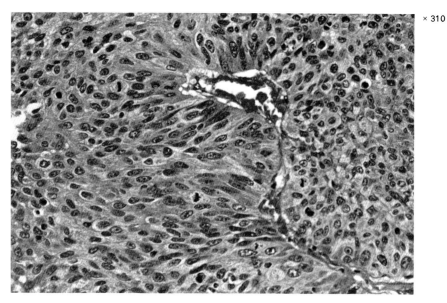

× 310

Fig. 24. " Transitional " carcinoma, nasal cavity
Nonkeratinizing respiratory-type epithelium with malignant cytological features. **Numerous mitoses.** Same case as Fig. 23

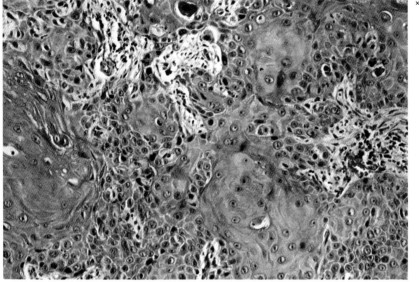

× 160

Fig. 25. Nasopharyngeal carcinoma — squamous cell carcinoma
Well differentiated. Keratinization and intercellular bridges

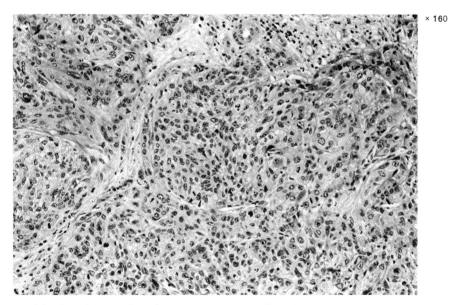

× 160

Fig. 26. Nasopharyngeal carcinoma — squamous cell carcinoma
Poorly differentiated. Minimal but definite evidence of squamous differentiation.

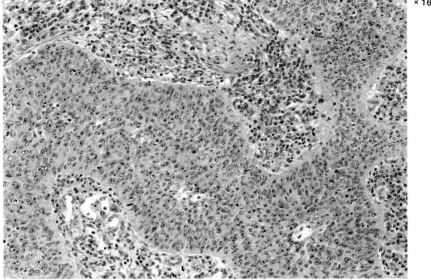

× 160

Fig. 27. Nasopharyngeal carcinoma — nonkeratinizing carcinoma
Well-defined plexiform masses of nonkeratinizing pavemented cells

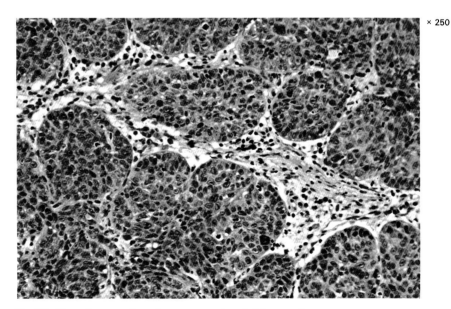

× 250

Fig. 28. Nasopharyngeal carcinoma — nonkeratinizing carcinoma
Well-defined masses of nonkeratinizing pavemented cells

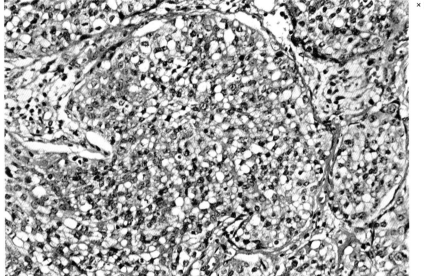

× 250

Fig. 29. Nasopharyngeal carcinoma — nonkeratinizing carcinoma
Clear cell structure

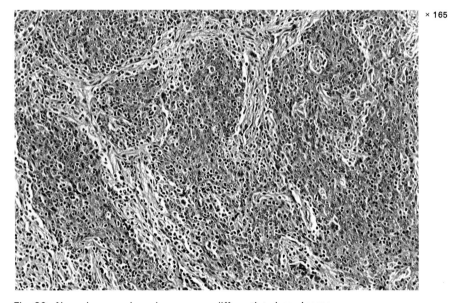

× 165

Fig. 30. Nasopharyngeal carcinoma — undifferentiated carcinoma
Lymphoepithelial carcinoma. Irregular masses of undifferentiated tumour cells heavily admixed with lymphocytes

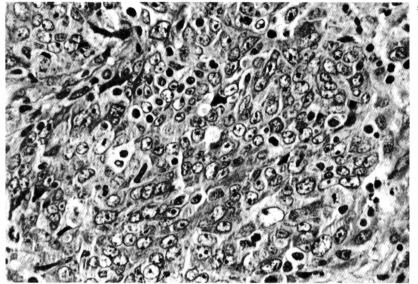

× 480

Fig. 31. Nasopharyngeal carcinoma — undifferentiated carcinoma
Tumour cells with vesicular nuclei admixed with lymphocytes. Syncytial structure

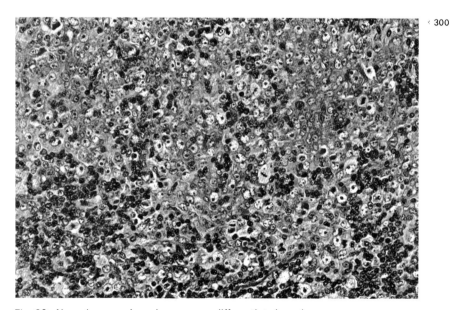

< 300

Fig. 32. Nasopharyngeal carcinoma — undifferentiated carcinoma
Syncytial appearance of undifferentiated tumour cells

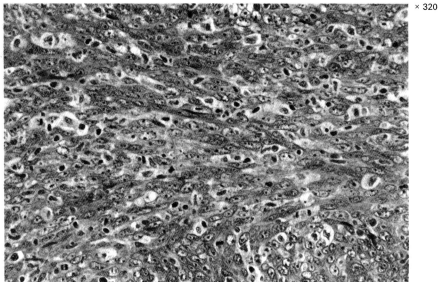

Fig. 33. Nasopharyngeal carcinoma — undifferentiated carcinoma
Spindle-shaped tumour cells

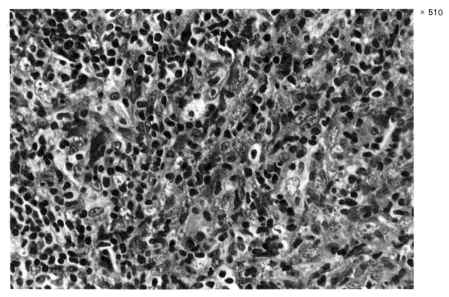

Fig. 34. Nasopharyngeal carcinoma — undifferentiated carcinoma
Loosely connected tumour cells in lymphoid stroma

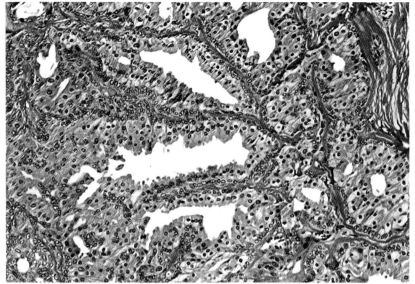

Fig. 35. Ceruminous adenoma, external auditory meatus
Glandular structure with bilayered epithelium

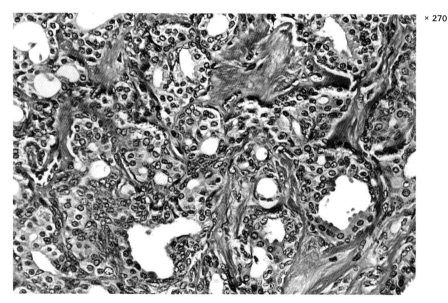

Fig. 36. Ceruminous adenoma, external auditory meatus
Glandular structure with fibrous stroma

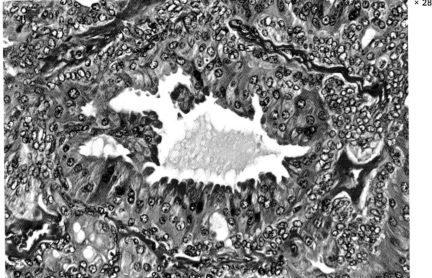

Fig. 37. Ceruminous adenoma, external auditory meatus
Oxyphilic tumour cells with apocrine features. Bilayered arrangement

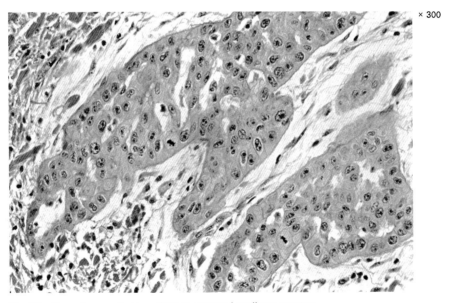

Fig. 38. Ceruminous adenocarcinoma, external auditory meatus
Poorly formed glandular structures. Mitoses and stromal invasion

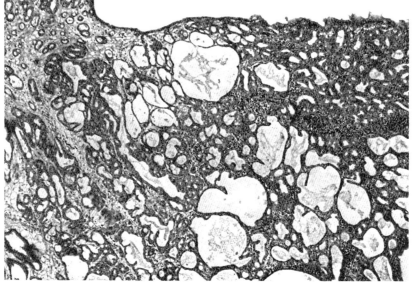

× 65

Fig. 39. Adenocarcinoma, nasopharynx
Well-differentiated tumour with close resemblance to adenoma

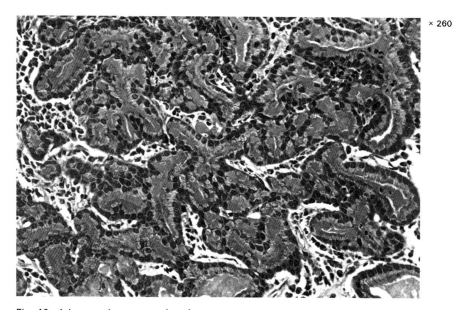

× 260

Fig. 40. Adenocarcinoma, nasal cavity
Tubular structure. Well-differentiated tumour with close resemblance to adenoma

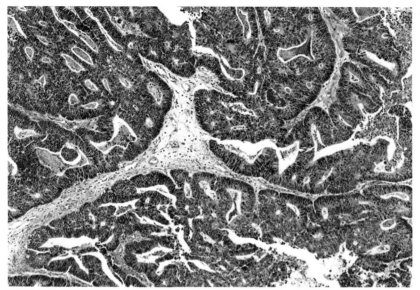

× 80

Fig. 41. Adenocarcinoma, maxillary sinus
Moderately differentiated

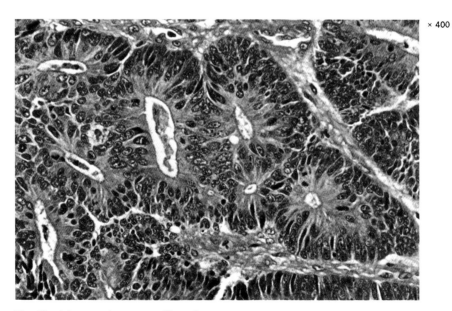

× 400

Fig. 42. Adenocarcinoma, maxillary sinus
Moderately differentiated. Same case as Fig. 41

× 160

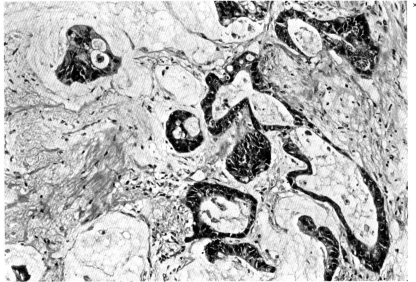

Fig. 43. Mucinous adenocarcinoma, ethmoid sinus
Irregular glandular structure. Lakes of extracellular mucus

× 250

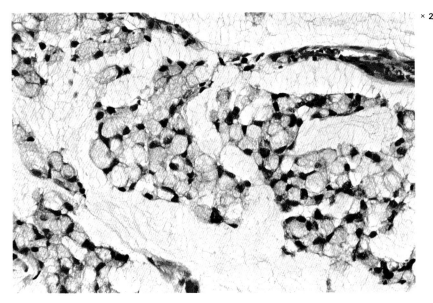

Fig. 44. Mucinous adenocarcinoma, maxillary sinus
Signet ring cells. Intracellular and extracellular mucus

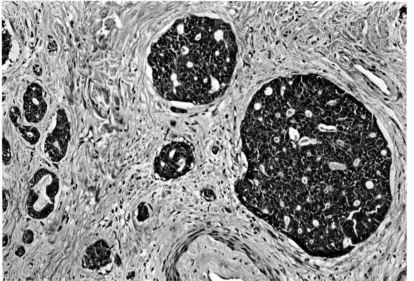

× 160

Fig. 45. Adenoid cystic carcinoma, maxillary sinus
Uniform small cells arranged in solid masses and duct-like structures

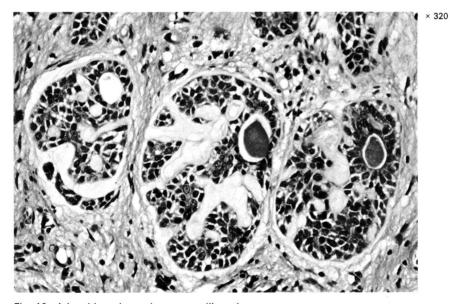

× 320

Fig. 46. Adenoid cystic carcinoma, maxillary sinus
Tumour masses with mucus-filled duct-like structures and hyaline mucoid material in stroma

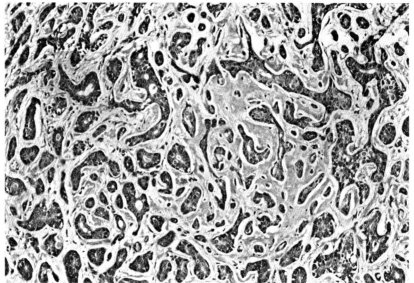

× 160

Fig. 47. Adenoid cystic carcinoma, maxillary sinus
Duct-like structures in fibrous stroma. Same case as Figs. 45 and 46

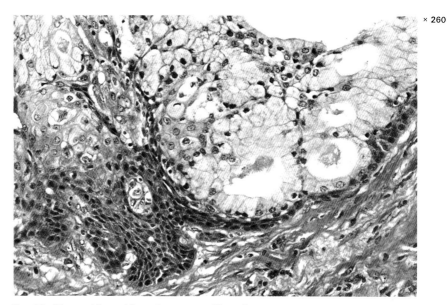

× 260

Fig. 48. Mucoepidermoid carcinoma, maxillary sinus
Multilayered squamous cells and glandular structures lined by mucus cells

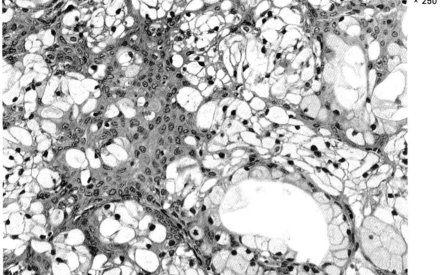

Fig. 49. Mucoepidermoid carcinoma, nasal cavity
Squamous cells, mucus cells, and cells with clear cytoplasm

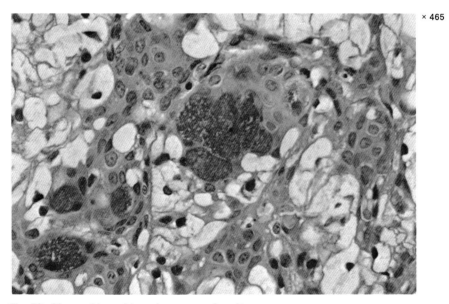

Fig. 50. Mucoepidermoid carcinoma, nasal cavity
Same case as Fig. 49. Mucicarmine

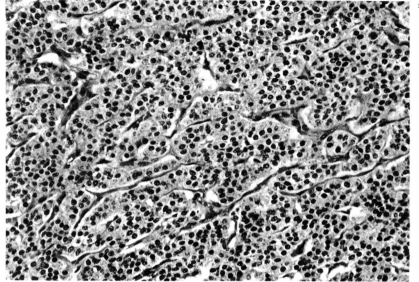

× 280

Fig. 51. Carcinoid tumour, trachea
Uniform cells with rounded nuclei and granular cytoplasm. Trabecular structure

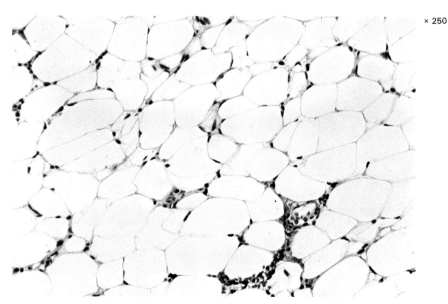

× 250

Fig. 52. Lipoma, hypopharynx
Mature adipose tissue cells

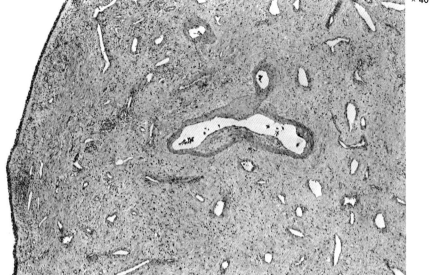

Fig. 53. Juvenile angiofibroma, nasopharynx
Thick- and thin-walled vessels in fibrous stroma. Focal intimal thickening

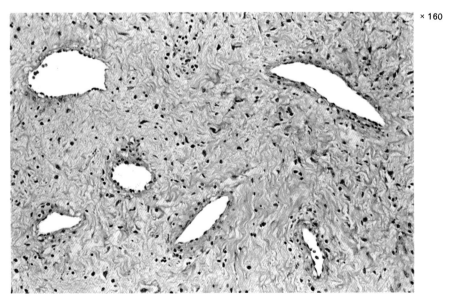

Fig. 54. Juvenile angiofibroma, nasopharynx
Thin-walled vessels in fibrous stroma

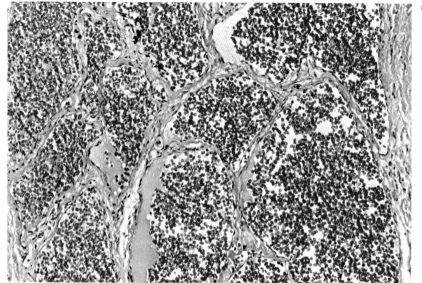

Fig. 55. Haemangioma, nasal cavity

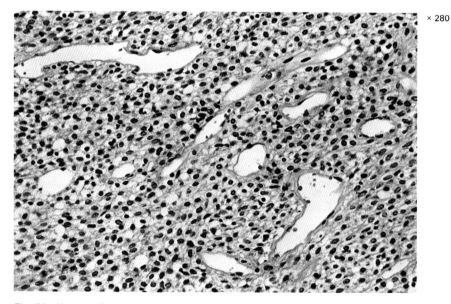

Fig. 56. Haemangiopericytoma, nasal cavity
Uniform tumour cells arranged about vascular spaces lined by single layer of endothelial cells

× 160

× 280

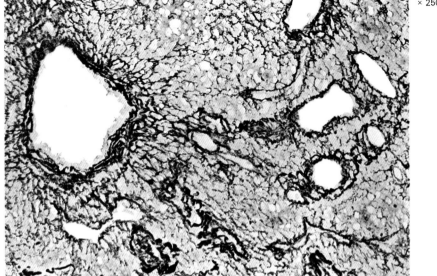

Fig. 57. Haemangiopericytoma, nasal cavity
Tumour cells surrounded by reticulin fibres and arranged about vascular spaces. Reticulin

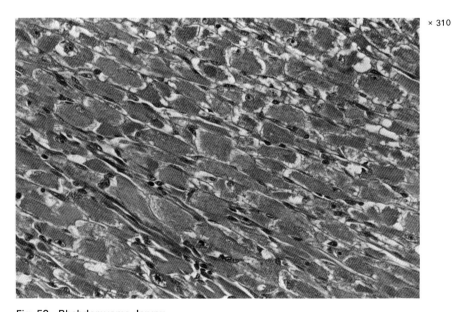

Fig. 58. Rhabdomyoma, larynx
Large cells with eosinophilic cytoplasm. Cytoplasmic vacuolation

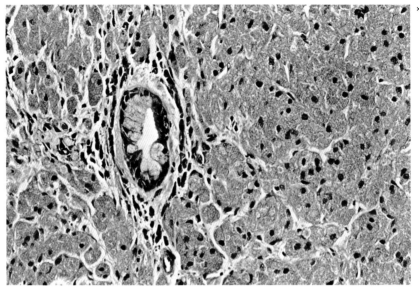

× 250

Fig. 59. Granular cell tumour, larynx
Tumour cells with pyknotic nuclei and abundant granular eosinophilic cytoplasm surrounding
a laryngeal gland

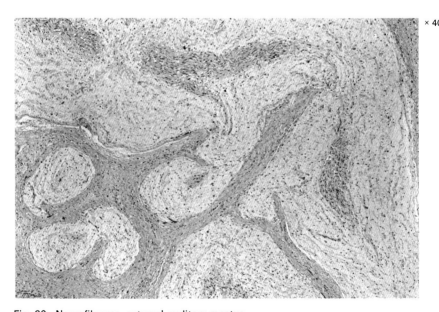

× 40

Fig. 60. Neurofibroma, external auditory meatus
Plexiform neurofibroma with growth of Schwann cells and fibroblasts around nerves

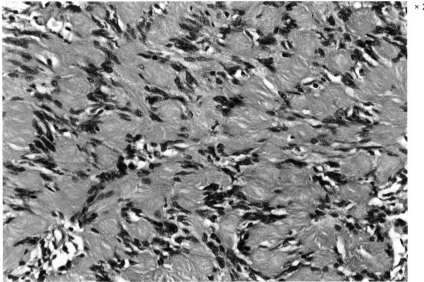

× 270

Fig. 61. Neurilemmoma, nasal cavity
Organoid pattern with palisading of nuclei. Antoni type A

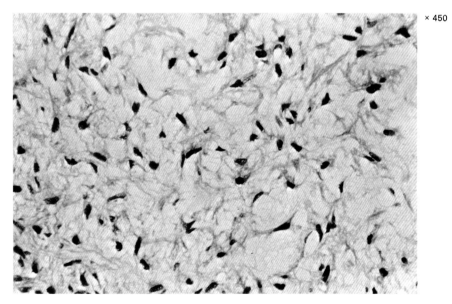

× 450

Fig. 62. Myxoma, nasal cavity
Spindle and stellate cells in a myxoid matrix

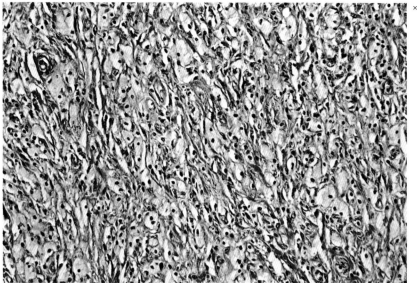

× 160

Fig. 63. Fibroxanthoma, nasal cavity
Histiocytes with foamy cytoplasm, fibroblasts and collagen fibres

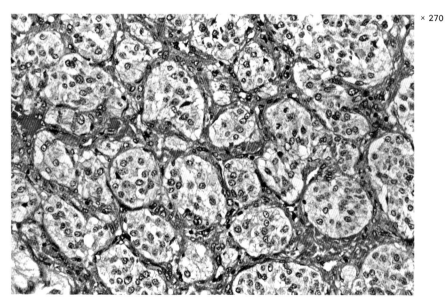

× 270

Fig. 64. Paraganglioma, middle ear
Nests of epithelioid tumour cells with finely granular cytoplasm in a vascular stroma

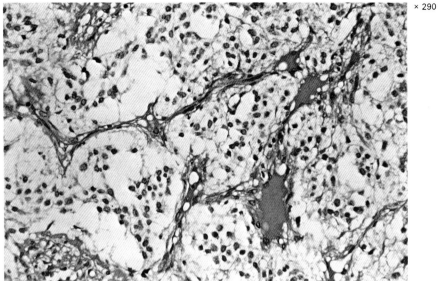

× 290

Fig. 65. Paraganglioma, middle ear
Tumour cells with moth-eaten appearance

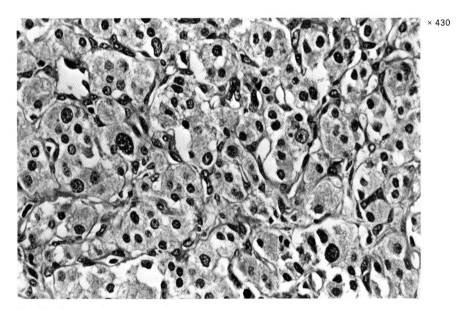

× 430

Fig. 66. Paraganglioma, nasopharynx
Moderate nuclear pleomorphism

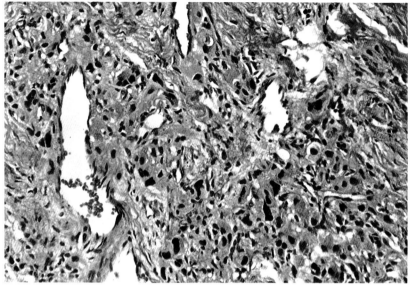

× 250

Fig. 67. Paraganglioma, middle ear
Nuclear hyperchromatism and pleomorphism. Stromal haemosiderin deposits. From a locally invasive tumour

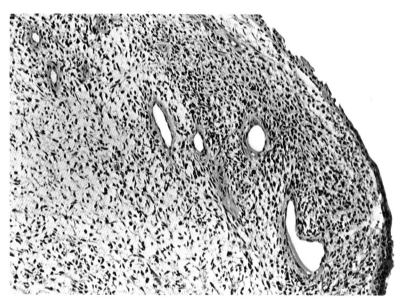

× 160

Fig. 68. Embryonal rhabdomyosarcoma, external auditory meatus
Tumour cells in myxoid matrix. Richly cellular zone close to epithelial surface

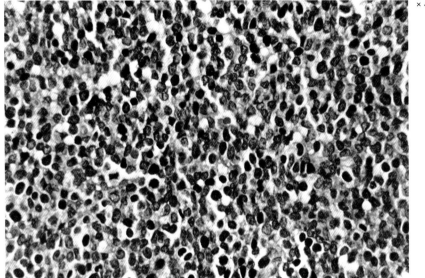

× 480

Fig. 69. Embryonal rhabdomyosarcoma, nasal cavity
Tumour cells with scanty cytoplasm

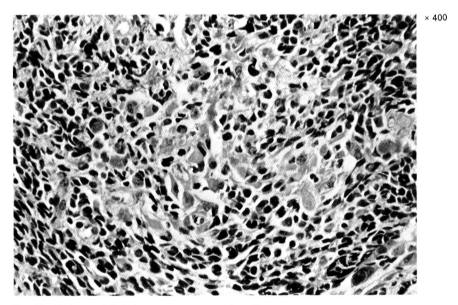

× 400

Fig. 70. Embryonal rhabdomyosarcoma, nasal cavity
Tumour cells with varying amounts of eosinophilic cytoplasm

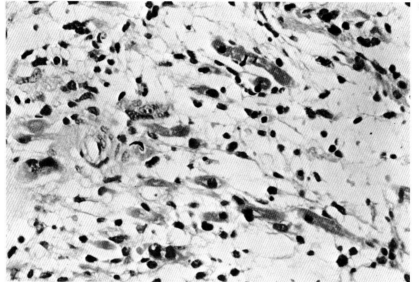

× 400

Fig. 71. Embryonal rhabdomyosarcoma, nasopharynx
Strap-like tumour cells with eosinophilic cytoplasm

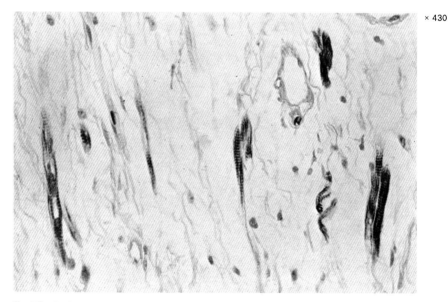

× 430

Fig. 72. Embryonal rhabdomyosarcoma, nasopharynx
Cross striations. Same case as Fig. 71. PTAH

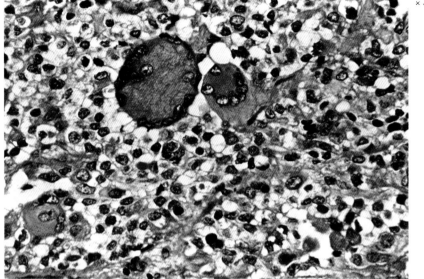

× 480

Fig. 73. Embryonal rhabdomyosarcoma, nasal cavity
Tumour cells with vacuolated cytoplasm. Two tumour giant cells with peripherally arranged nuclei

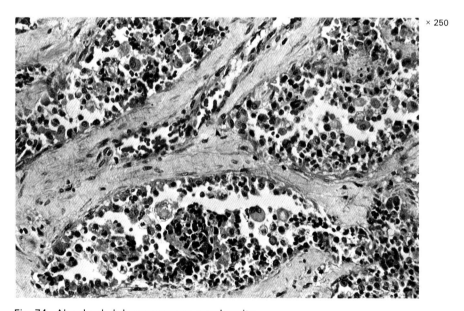

× 250

Fig. 74. Alveolar rhabdomyosarcoma, nasal cavity
Tumour cells arranged in well-defined alveolar masses

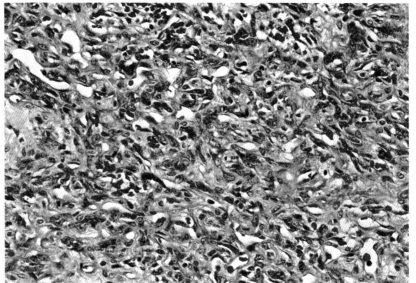

× 280

Fig. 75. Angiosarcoma, nasopharynx
Irregular vascular channels lined by malignant endothelial cells

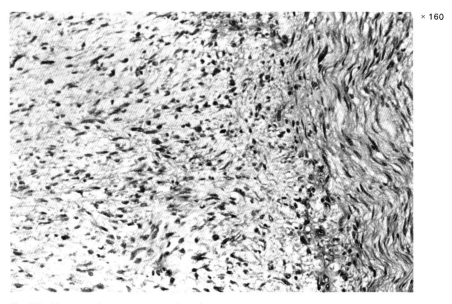

× 160

Fig. 76. Neurogenic sarcoma, nasal cavity
Spindle-celled sarcomatous tumour occurring in relation to a nerve trunk

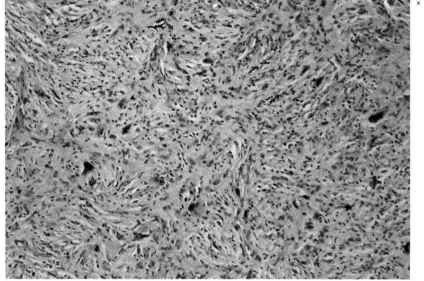

× 100

Fig. 77. Malignant fibroxanthoma, maxillary sinus

Histiocytic and fibroblast-like tumour cells, some bizarre and multinucleated, in storiform arrangement

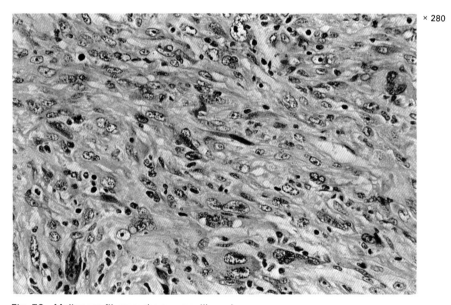

× 280

Fig. 78. Malignant fibroxanthoma, maxillary sinus

Histiocytic and fibroblast-like tumour cells with foamy cytoplasm. Chronic inflammatory cells

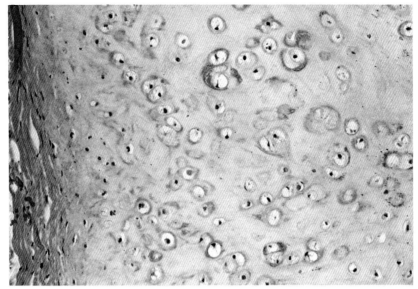

Fig. 79. Chondroma, larynx
Mature cartilage cells

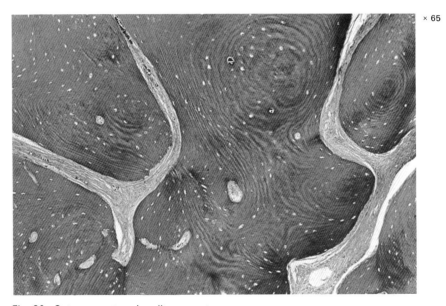

Fig. 80. Osteoma, external auditory meatus
Mature bone with lamellar structure

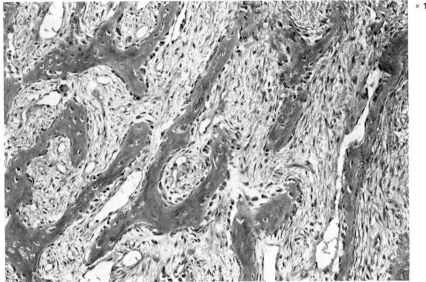

×160

Fig. 81. Ossifying fibroma, maxilla
Fibroblastic tissue with spicules of metaplastic bone rimmed by osteoblasts

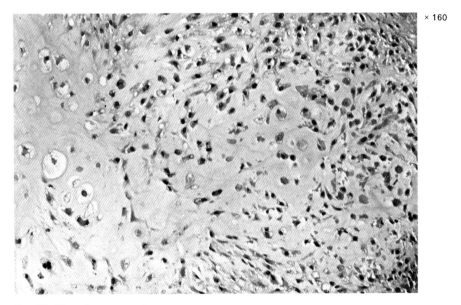

×160

Fig. 82. Chondrosarcoma, larynx
Cartilaginous tumour with atypia and increased cellularity

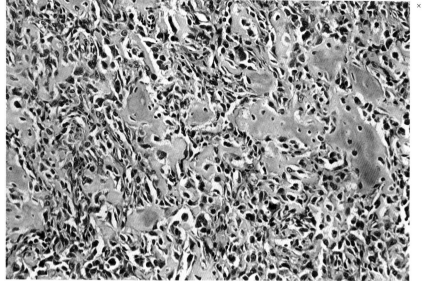

×160

Fig. 83. Osteosarcoma, maxilla
Osteoid formation by tumour cells

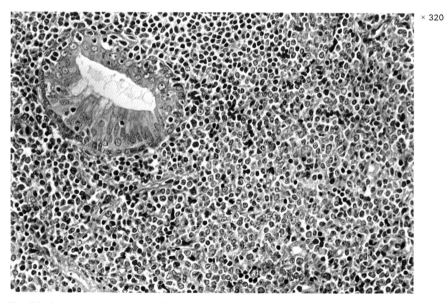

×320

Fig. 84. Lymphosarcoma, nasopharynx

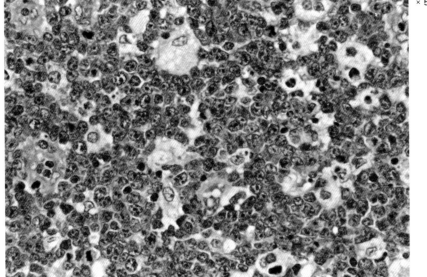

× 510

Fig. 85. Burkitt's tumour, maxillary sinus

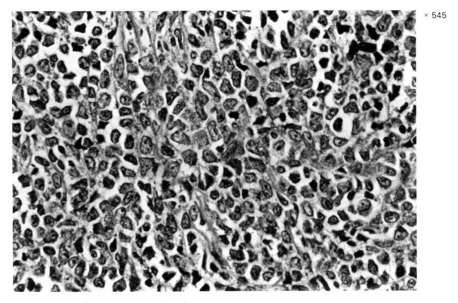

× 545

Fig. 86. Reticulosarcoma, nasal cavity

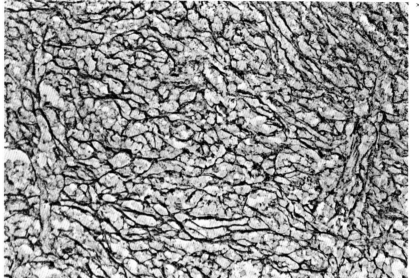

×270

Fig. 87. Reticulosarcoma, nasal cavity
Same case as Fig. 86. Reticulin

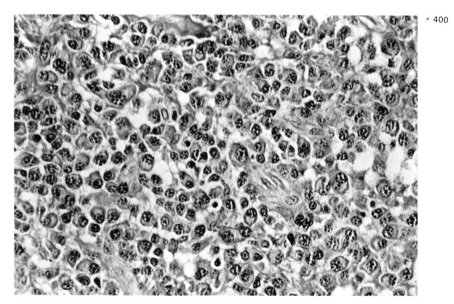

×400

Fig. 88. Plasmacytoma, nasopharynx

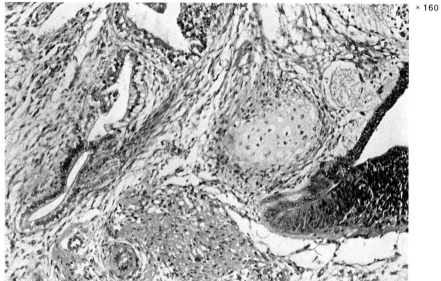

× 160

Fig. 89. Teratoma, nasal cavity
Mature and immature tissues

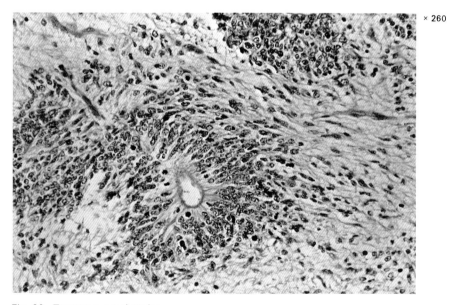

× 260

Fig. 90. Teratoma, nasal cavity
Immature neurogenic tissue. Same case as Fig. 89

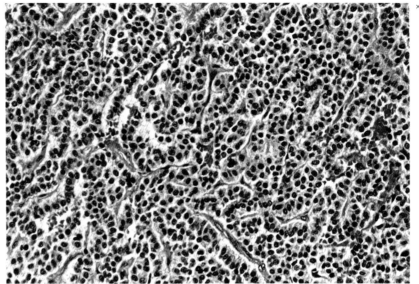

× 290

Fig. 91. Pituitary adenoma, nasopharynx
Columns of polygonal cells with regular nuclei and amphophilic cytoplasm, separated by thin-walled vascular channels

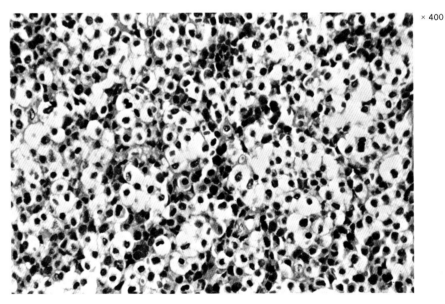

× 400

Fig. 92. Pituitary adenoma, nasopharynx
Nests of acidophilic and clear cells. Same case as Fig. 91

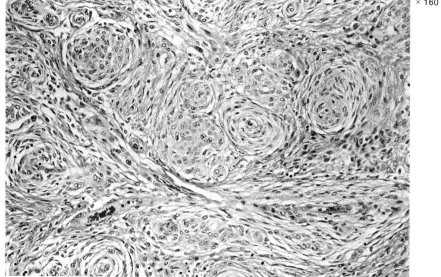
× 160

Fig. 93. Meningioma, nasal cavity
Nests and perivascular whorls of meningothelial cells

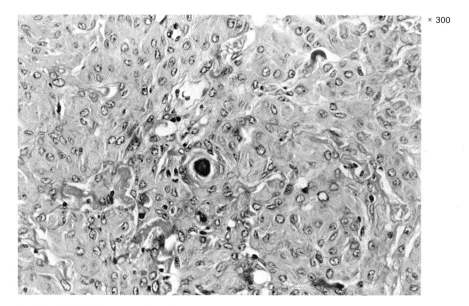
× 300

Fig. 94. Meningioma, nasal cavity
Psammoma body among meningothelial cells

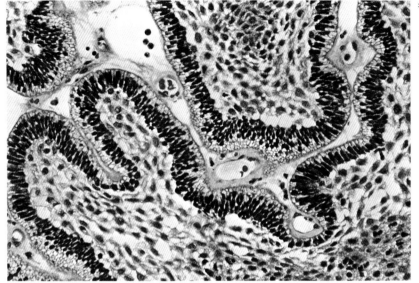

Fig. 95. Ameloblastoma, maxillary sinus
Tumour masses, with central stellate and peripheral columnar cells

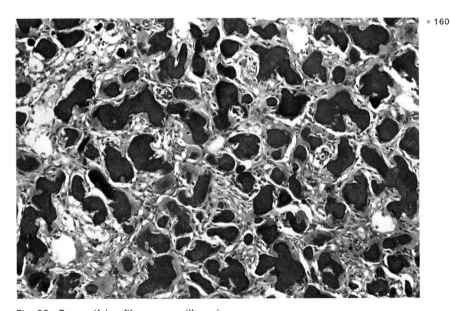

Fig. 96. Cementifying fibroma, maxillary sinus
Calcified masses of cementum-like tissue separated by fibroblastic cells

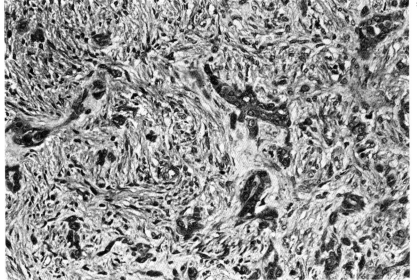

× 160

Fig. 97. Melanotic neuroectodermal tumour, maxilla
Duct-like structures and strands of epithelial cells in a cellular fibrous stroma

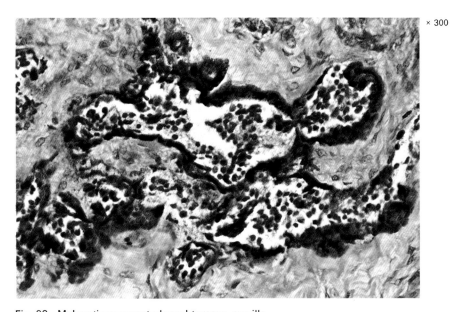

× 300

Fig. 98. Melanotic neuroectodermal tumour, maxilla
Irregular space containing small neuroblast-like cells lined by heavily pigmented epithelial cells. Fibrous stroma

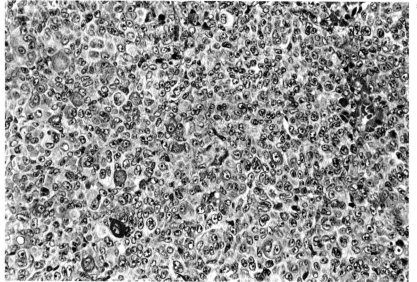

Fig. 99. Malignant melanoma, nasal cavity
Tumour cells with melanin pigment

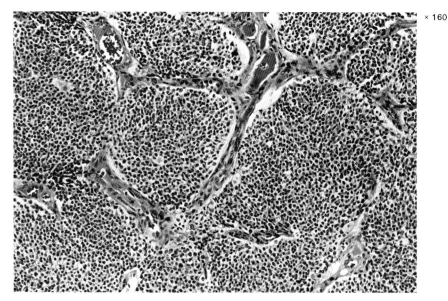

Fig. 100. Olfactory neurogenic tumour, nasal cavity
Esthesioneurocytoma. Lobular architecture

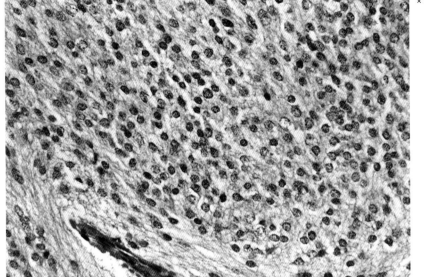

× 300

Fig. 101. Olfactory neurogenic tumour, nasal cavity
Esthesioneurocytoma. Uniform neurocytes and neurofibrils

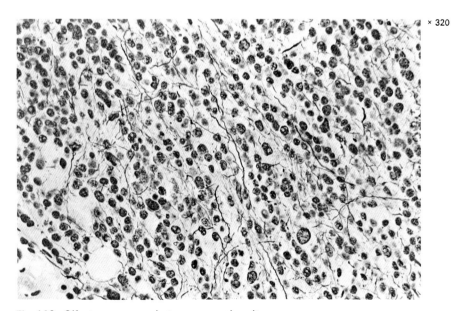

× 320

Fig. 102. Olfactory neurogenic tumour, nasal cavity
Esthesioneurocytoma. Neurofibrils. Bodian

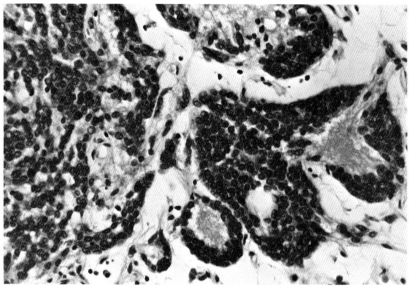

× 300

Fig. 103. Olfactory neurogenic tumour, nasal cavity

Esthesioneurocytoma. Pseudorosettes with masses of eosinophilc fibrils surrounded by uniform tumour cells

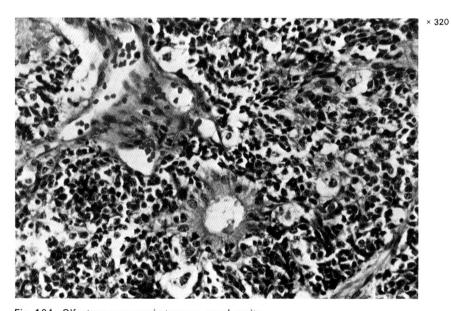

× 320

Fig. 104. Olfactory neurogenic tumour, nasal cavity

Esthesioneuroepithelioma. Rosette formation with columnar cells lining a clearly defined central cavity

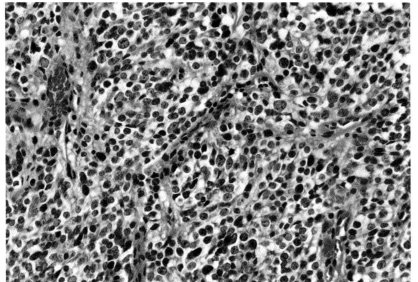

× 320

Fig. 105. Olfactory neurogenic tumour, nasal cavity
Esthesioneuroblastoma. Cellular pleomorphism

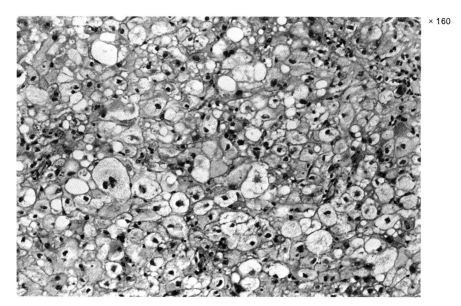

× 160

Fig. 106. Chordoma, nasopharynx
Large, pleomorphic cells with prominent cell membranes and voluminous vacuolated cytoplasm

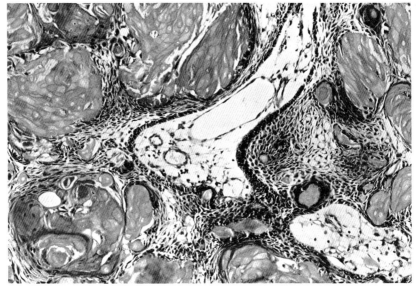

Fig. 107. Craniopharyngioma, nasopharynx
Prominent keratinisation

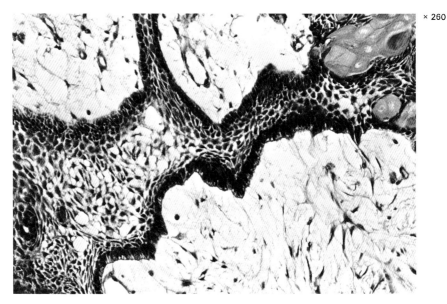

Fig. 108. Craniopharyngioma, nasopharynx
Branching masses of stellate epithelial cells with palisaded columnar cells at periphery.
Oedematous stroma

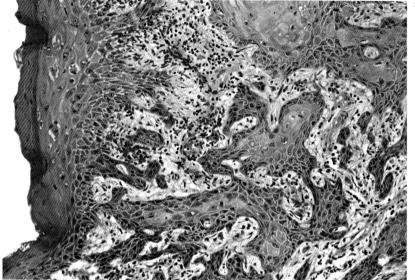

Fig. 109. Pseudoepitheliomatous hyperplasia, nasal cavity
Irregular downgrowth of mature squamous epithelium

× 160

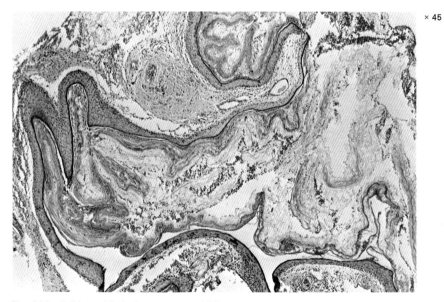

Fig. 110. Epidermoid cholesteatoma, middle ear
Well-differentiated squamous epithelium lining cavity containing laminated masses of keratin

× 45

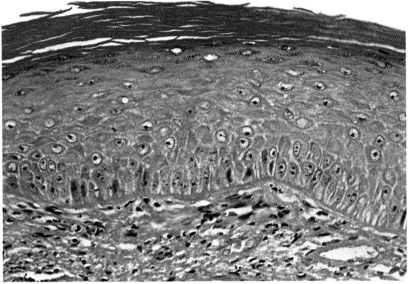

× 300

Fig. 111. Keratosis, larynx
Excessive keratin formation

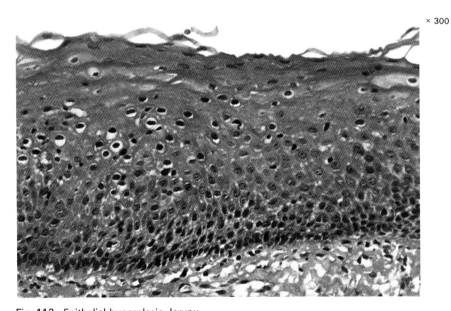

× 300

Fig. 112. Epithelial hyperplasia, larynx
Increase in cell layers

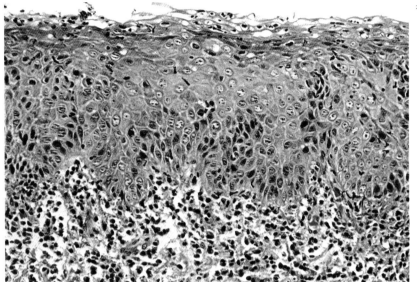

Fig. 113. Dysplasia, larynx
Moderate cellular atypia with partial loss of normal stratification

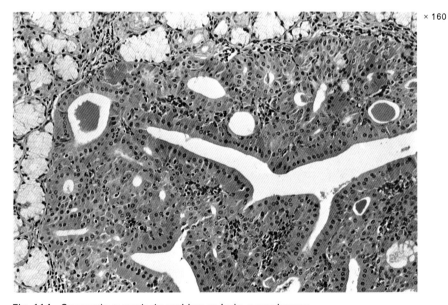

Fig. 114. Oncocytic metaplasia and hyperplasia, nasopharynx
Metaplastic cells with abundant eosinophilic cytoplasm and normal mucous glands

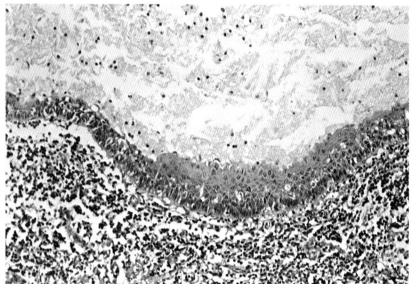

× 250

Fig. 115. Cyst, nasopharynx
    Cyst lined by squamous and respiratory-type epithelium

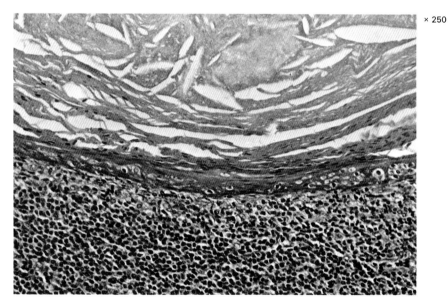

× 250

Fig. 116. Cyst, nasopharynx
    Keratin-filled cyst lined by stratified squamous epithelium

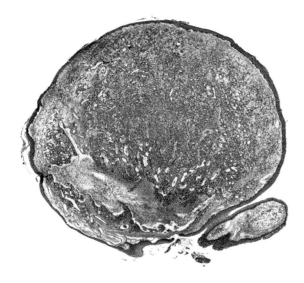

Fig. 117. Angiogranuloma, nasal cavity
Polypoid lesion consisting of richly vascular tissue

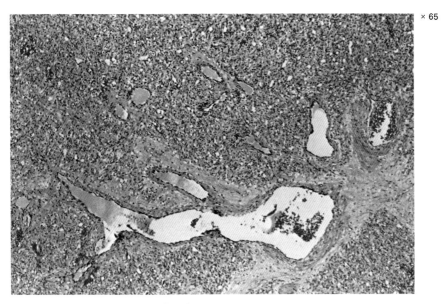

Fig. 118. Angiogranuloma, nasal cavity
Masses of capillaries supplied by muscular arteries

× 300

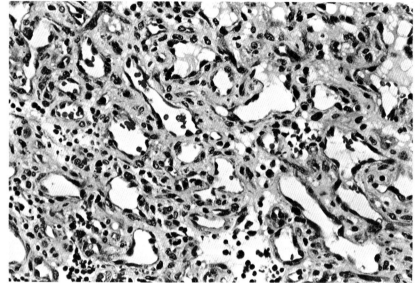

Fig. 119. Angiogranuloma, nasal cavity
Capillaries separated by stroma containing inflammatory cells

× 160

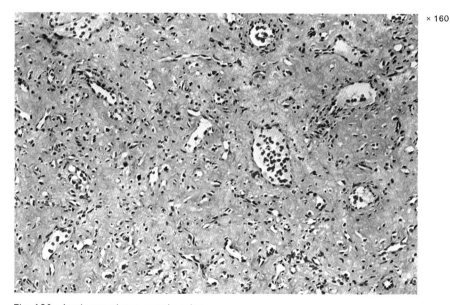

Fig. 120. Angiogranuloma, nasal cavity
Capillaries separated by fibrous stroma

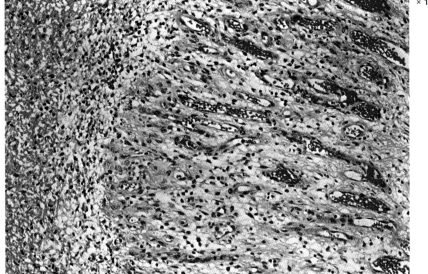

× 160

Fig. 121. Intubation granuloma, larynx
Vascular granulation tissue

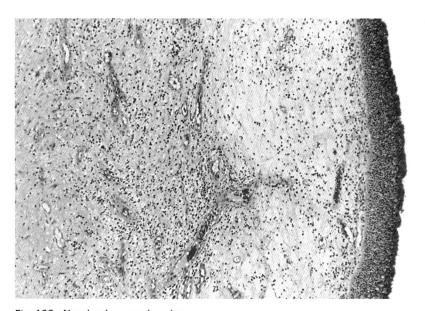

× 75

Fig. 122. Nasal polyp, nasal cavity
Oedematous nasal mucosa infiltrated by inflammatory cells

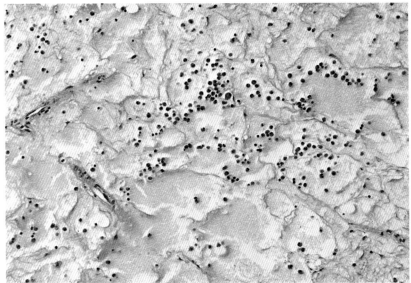

× 160

Fig. 123. Nasal polyp, nasal cavity
Stromal oedema and infiltration by eosinophils

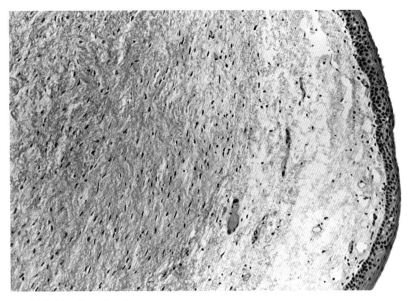

× 160

Fig. 124. Vocal cord polyp
Fibrous polyp

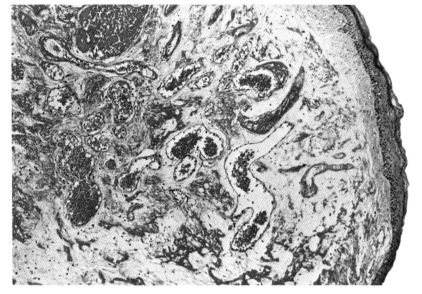

× 75

Fig. 125. Vocal cord polyp
Hyaline, vascular polyp

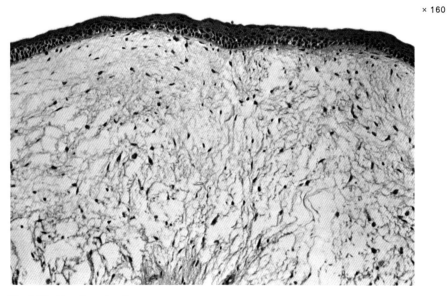

× 160

Fig. 126. Vocal cord polyp
Myxoid polyp

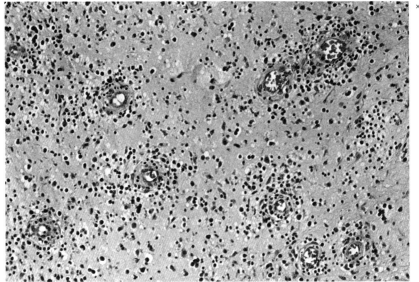

×160

Fig. 127. Otic polyp, external auditory meatus
Oedematous granulation tissue with infiltration by inflammatory cells

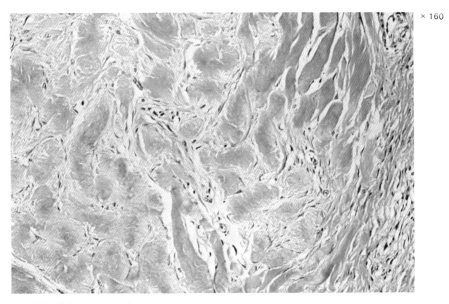

×160

Fig. 128. Keloid, external ear
Broad, interlacing eosinophilic bands of collagen

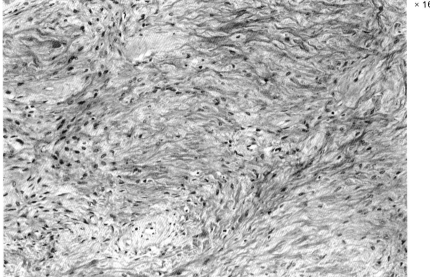

× 160

Fig. 129. Fibromatosis, nasal cavity
Fibroblasts with abundant collagen formation

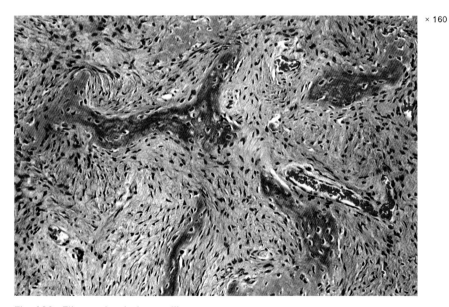

× 160

Fig. 130. Fibrous dysplasia, maxilla
Fibrous connective tissue with islands of non-lamellar metaplastic bone

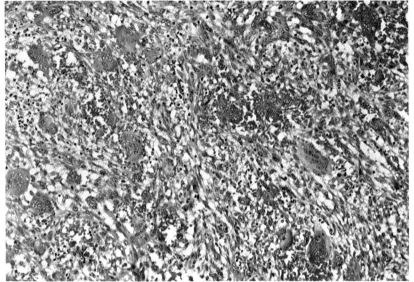

× 160

Fig. 131. Giant cell " reparative " granuloma, maxilla
Aggregates of multinucleated giant cells in fibroblastic tissue

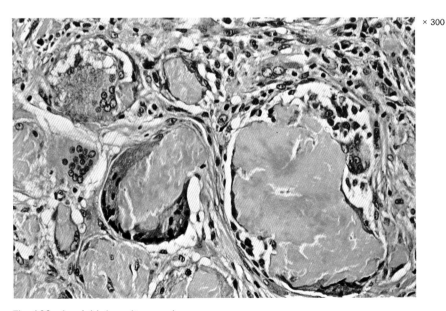

× 300

Fig. 132. Amyloid deposit, nasopharynx
Hyaline masses of amyloid with foreign body giant cells

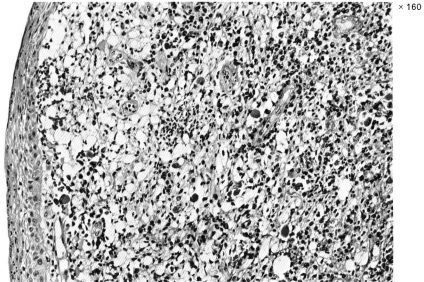

× 160

Fig. 133. Rhinoscleroma, nasal cavity
Large vacuolated macrophages and plasma cells. Several Russell bodies

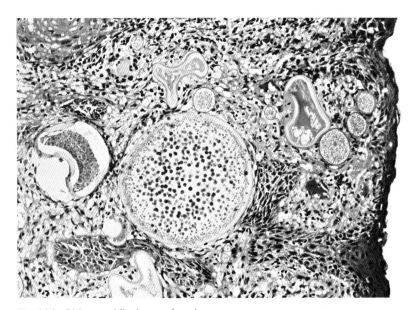

× 160

Fig. 134. Rhinosporidiosis, nasal cavity
Sporangia in various stages of development containing spores of *Rhinosporidium seeberi*

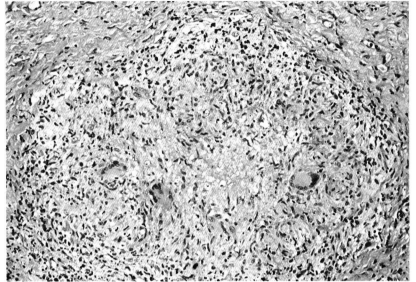

× 160

Fig. 135. Tuberculosis, larynx
Granulomatous lesion with epithelioid histiocytes and Langhans' giant cells

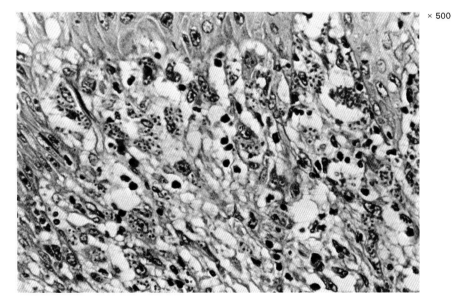

× 500

Fig. 136. Histoplasmosis, larynx
Histoplasma capsulatum within macrophages. PAS

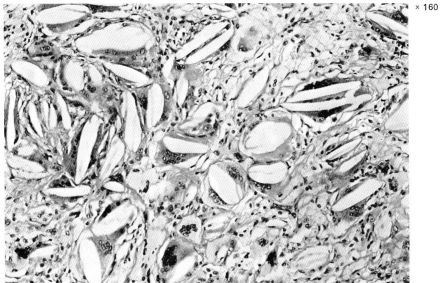

× 160

Fig. 137. Cholesterol granuloma, middle ear
Cholesterol clefts bounded by foreign body giant cells

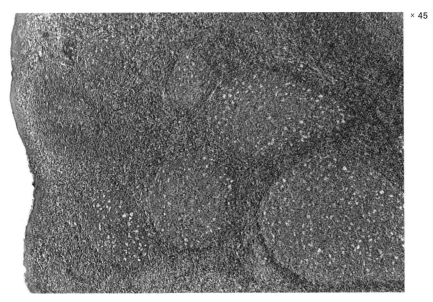

× 45

Fig. 138. Benign lymphoid hyperplasia, nasopharynx
Lymphoid follicles with large germinal centres

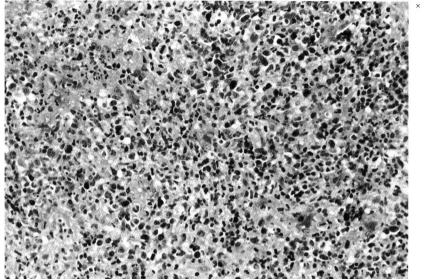

× 280

Fig. 139. Lethal midline granuloma, nasopharynx
Pleomorphic cellular infiltrate

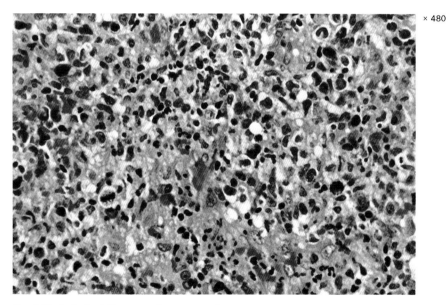

× 480

Fig. 140. Lethal midline granuloma, nasopharynx
Histiocytes with abnormal nuclei and mitoses admixed with neutrophils and lymphocytes

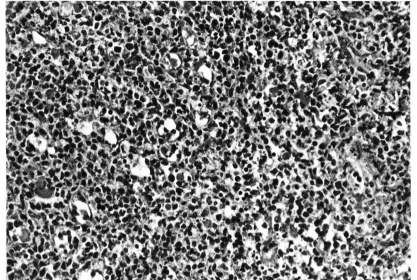

×310

Fig. 141. Lethal midline granuloma, nasal cavity
Immature lymphoid cells and histiocytes

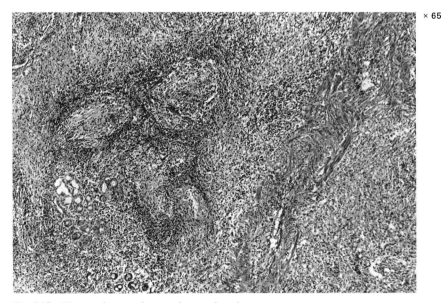

×65

Fig. 142. Wegener's granulomatosis, nasal cavity
Vasculitis and granulomatous inflammation

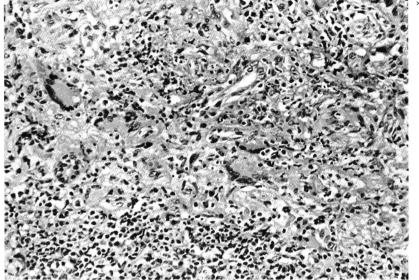

× 270

Fig. 143. Wegener's granulomatosis, nasal cavity
Granulomatous lesion with giant cells

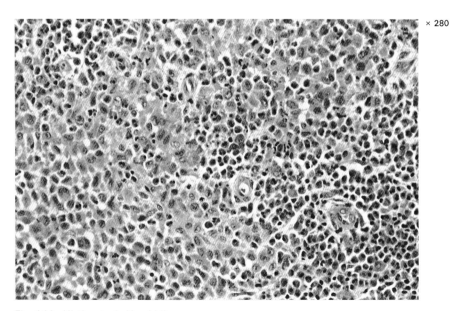

× 280

Fig. 144. Histiocytosis X, middle ear
Mature histiocytes and eosinophils

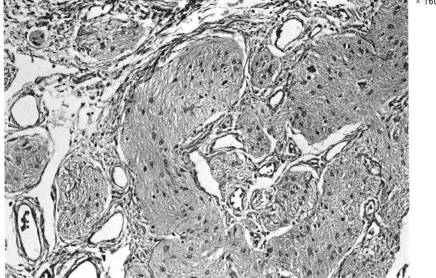

× 160

Fig. 145. Nasal glial heterotopia, nasal cavity
Masses of mature astrocytes and glial fibres

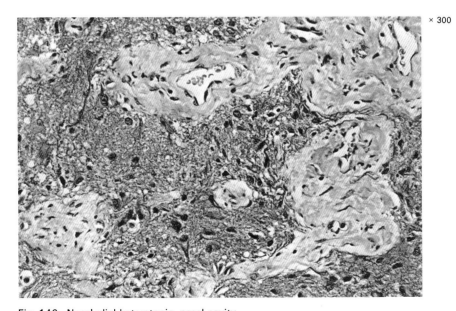

× 300

Fig. 146. Nasal glial heterotopia, nasal cavity
Protoplasmic astrocytes in meshwork of glial fibres. Fibrous stroma. PTAH

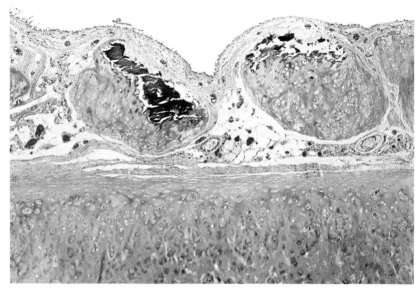

Fig. 147. Tracheopathia osteochondroplastica
Submucous nodules of calcifying cartilage

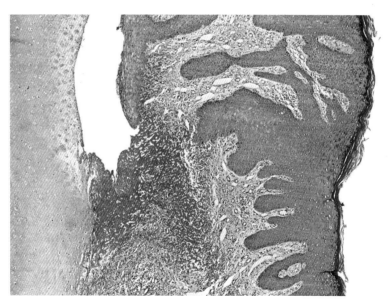

Fig. 148. Chondrodermatitis nodularis chronica helicis
Perichondrial inflammation with fibrinoid exudate and cyst formation

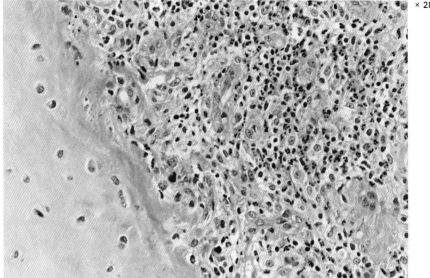

Fig. 149. Chondrodermatitis nodularis chronica helicis
Perichondrial inflammation

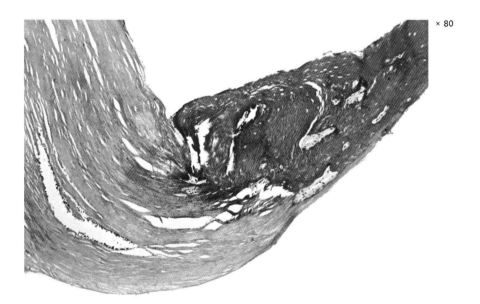

Fig. 150. Tympanosclerosis, middle ear
Hyalinized fibrous tissue with bone formation